The
COUNTRY VET'S

Home
Remedies
for
Dogs

Kim Campbell Thornton

Consultant: William Fortney, D.V.M.

Publications International, Ltd.

Kim Campbell Thornton is former editor of *Dog Fancy* magazine and has numerous books to her credit, including *For the Love of Dogs*, *Why Do Dogs Do That?*, and *Dog Treats*. She frequently contributes articles to *Veterinary Practice Staff*, the *AKC Gazette*, and *Dogs USA*. A member of the Dog Writers Association of America, she serves on its Board of Governors and on the board of the Dog Writers Educational Trust.

William Fortney, D.V.M., is a professor of veterinary medicine and director of community practice service at the Veterinary Medical Teaching Hospital of Kansas State University. His specialties include preventative medicine, infectious diseases, and pediatric and geriatric medicine. Dr. Fortney has served as president of the Kansas Veterinary Medical Association, was named Kansas "Veterinarian of the Year," and has been appointed to the Kansas Pet Advisory Board.

Editorial Assistance: David Kay

Illustrations: Barbara Emmons

Cover photo: **Zack Burris, Inc.**

Louis Weber, C.E.O.
Publications International, Ltd.
7373 North Cicero Avenue
Lincolnwood, Illinois 60646

Permission is never granted for commercial purposes.

Manufactured in China.

8 7 6 5 4 3 2 1

ISBN: 0-7853-2449-6

Library of Congress Catalog Card Number: 97-75513

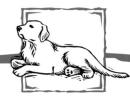

CONTENTS

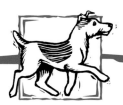

INTRODUCTION

I've loved dogs all my life, ever since I was a little boy growing up in the country. We always had dogs, and they were my best friends. Not just because we had so many good times together—fishing, swimming, roaming the hills—but because my parents taught me to respect and care for animals. Like all smart country people, they knew the more effort you put into animals, the more they gave back, whether it was eggs from a hen, milk from a cow, or the love and guardianship of a dog.

The values I learned about dog care were simple enough—feed them well, keep them clean, teach them manners, care for them when they're sick—but they made a big impression on me. If animals were that important, I wanted to spend my life caring for them. That's why I became a veterinarian.

As I grew older, I started to see just how and why dogs added so much to people's lives. Dogs bring us a lot of benefits—some that are clear as day and others we might not even notice. Why, even just talking to a dog makes most folks feel better. In my veterinary practice, I've learned that lots of people talk to their dogs. They talk to them about what's going on in their lives, their joys, their sorrows, even about problems they're having at work or school. Do the dogs talk back? Not yet, but they do something better: They listen. Unlike people, dogs listen intently to everything we have to say. Dogs provide a nonjudgmental ear—a sounding board, if you will—something that all of us could use in our daily lives.

Dogs are good for our health, too. If you want to have a long life with fewer doctor visits, here are some tips, straight from the horse's mouth: Eat right, exercise, and get a dog. All kinds of studies have shown that dog owners have lower blood pressure and cholesterol levels and fewer minor health problems than people without pets. Coronary patients who own dogs are much less likely to die within one year of hospitalization than those who don't own dogs.

Another way dogs keep us healthy is by providing stress relief. When we become stressed, our blood pressure and heart rate increase, we breathe faster, and our bodies receive a burst of hormones. All of these reactions are the body's attempt to help us deal with the situation. But too often we bottle up these responses, allowing hormones to build up and nervous system rates to remain high, a situation that can burden the body and damage the cardiovascular system. Fortunately, stroking a dog, or even just being in the same room with one, can reduce harmful responses to stressful situations. Why? Researchers say it's because of the dog's nonjudgmental support.

Dogs improve our social lives. A dog is the best kind of icebreaker. She has no qualms about going up to strangers, canine or human, and saying, "Hi." And people are more likely to stop and chat when you have a dog. If they have a dog, too, it's an instant bond. Dogs have even served as matchmakers. I can't tell you how many of my patients have told me their dogs introduced them to their spouses. What better way to check out a prospective mate! Dogs are famous for their ability to judge character.

Bored with your life? Need to shed a few pounds? A dog is the perfect motivator. No matter what kind of dog you have, from a tiny Chihuahua to a massive Mastiff, there's some kind of activity or competition in which you can become involved. With a dog, you can enter dog shows, herding competitions, and obedience trials. You can go to training class, flyball games, and Frisbee flying disc contests. Or you can just go for a walk or run around the block. A dog gets you off your duff and out into the world.

The best buddy in the world is a dog. Whether the two of you are hanging out on the sofa watching television or on a road trip, a dog is always there. She doesn't argue about which TV show to watch or keep reminding you for 200 miles about the wrong turn you made at Nashville. Instead, she snuggles next to you, happy to bask in the glow of your presence.

The greatest thing of all about a dog is her everlasting capacity to give love. A dog's keen observational skills tell her when we're happy and when we're sad or mad. And when we're unhappy, a dog does her darndest to make us feel better. Dogs don't care what we look like, how much money we make, or what kind of house we live in. All that matters is that we share their lives. Dogs don't do a lot of the jobs they used to on the farm and ranch, but there's one job at which they can't be beat: That of friend.

If you are ready to make friends with a dog, this book will be your guide. You won't find any big, fancy words in it, but you will find a lot of plain old common sense—things that I learned growing up and things that I've learned in my years as a dog doctor.

You'll find helpful advice on choosing just the right dog for the life you lead as well as caring for her from puppyhood through old age. Starting with what you want and need from a dog—not to mention what a dog wants and needs from you—we'll talk about how to find a breeder or adopt a dog from a shelter, how to feed and care for your dog, and how to recognize common illnesses and get them taken care of before they become serious.

Each chapter contains easy-to-understand information about what to look for in a dog, how dogs behave and learn, grooming, nutrition, vaccinations, first aid, and more. Whenever possible, I've given advice to help you care for your dog at home, but that doesn't mean I'm trying to put myself or any other veterinarians out of business. No matter how much you love and care for your dog, some things just need to be handled by a professional. My recommendations tell you when your pet can safely be treated at home and when to call in the expert—your veterinarian.

Of course, with good home care and preventive veterinary medicine, you might not ever need the chapters on first aid and illness, but they are there just in case. I hope you'll find this book to be a basic reference that you'll use again and again.

One last thing: *The Country Vet's Home Remedies for Dogs* is not meant as a substitute for professional veterinary medical care or advice. The remedies and advice in this book have been checked with practicing veterinarians and animal care experts, but your own vet should be the final authority.

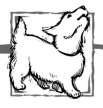

FIRST STEPS

I can always tell when a dog and his owner
are a good match. Just like a good match in
a marriage, they get to know each other's
ways, look out for one another, and even get
to looking like each other. Heck, it's almost
as if they can read each other's mind. Of
course, that's not always the case—some
people and their dogs are always scrapping
at each other. Somehow, something doesn't
quite fit right, and it shows.

That's why I always tell folks not to rush into
the relationship. Think about how a new dog
is going to change your life. He's going to
take up your time and energy with feeding,
grooming, exercise, and play. Dogs are smart,
social animals, so no matter what kind of dog
you get, he'll want and need to spend quality
time with you.

SHOULD I GET A PUPPY?

Now most people think starting off with a puppy is the best choice, but that isn't necessarily so. Raising a puppy is a labor-intensive undertaking, and it may take as long as three years for him to fully mature. Do you have young children or a full-time job? You might discover an adult dog is a better idea. You see, the best way to make sure you and your dog get off to the right start is to match up the pooch and his needs to you and your lifestyle.

No two puppies are exactly alike. Oh, some purebred litter mates may look as identical as peas in a pod, but rest assured they'll have their own individual personalities. Even if a particular breed is known for a certain kind of temperament, that's just a general trait. Each puppy will develop according to his own personality, which will also be affected by how the pup is raised and what the parents are like. In other words, you can't judge a book by its cover... and you can't judge a puppy solely by its breed or looks. If this were the case, you could get the perfect dog by mail order. Instead, you've got to take your time and use your head—and your heart—to make sure the dog you bring into your home is a good match.

It's probably a good idea to start looking at puppies a few weeks before you're ready to take one home. Remember, this is a long-term relationship (lifelong, for the dog). If you find the perfect puppy on the first try, that's great, but most people have to kiss a few canine frogs before they find their four-legged Prince or Princess Charming. Don't let sudden infatuation make the decision for you: Take a good look at him for signs of physical problems. A clean bill of health at this early age is the good start you want to make sure your new friend stays with you for a good long time. Here are some clues to look for:

- The eyes and nose should be clear and clean, not red or runny.

- The puppy's coat should be clear and shiny.

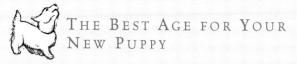

THE BEST AGE FOR YOUR NEW PUPPY

Puppies are born helpless. Their eyes and ears are closed, and their entire daily schedule consists of nursing and sleeping. By the age of about 14 days, their eyes and ears open, and they begin processing the world of light and sound. At three to four weeks of age, pups start to learn the serious business of play. They're mobile now, and familiar signs of canine communication like tail wags, yips, and yelps accompany their interactions with mom, the world, and each other. From this point until around 14 weeks is called the critical behavior period; this is when dogs form most of the foundation for their lifelong behavior. Contact with litter mates, mom, and—in small doses—humans is crucial during the critical period to ensure proper socialization. That's why the old practice of sending puppies to new homes by themselves at age seven or eight weeks has fallen out of favor. Between age two to three months seems to be the earliest a puppy is ready to start a new life with a loving family.

- Check the puppy's belly. All pups tend to be a little potbellied when they have a full tummy, but a puppy with a noticeably swollen belly has a good chance of harboring worms.

- Check for discharge from the rear end and chronic coughing and sneezing.

If you're an old softie like me, you'll probably want to take the runt of the litter home, complete with all his frailties. Be forewarned, though—a sickly puppy is more likely to have major health problems into adulthood, and veterinary bills can add up quickly. If you're not sure you can take on the added expense of a more needy dog, don't. There are far more healthy puppies in the world than there are good homes for them, so you'll be doing any puppy a favor by adopting him.

Evaluating a pup's personality is mostly a commonsense call. There's a very good chance a bright, friendly puppy will grow up to be a bright, friendly dog, and the timid pup cowering in the corner will continue to be shy. If you buy from a breeder, you have the right to expect the puppies to be well socialized and even accustomed to children, other pets in the household, and visitors to the home. The right amount of handling, exposure to a variety of sounds and scents, and the experience of life with humans, go a long way in setting your little pooch on the road to being a friendly, well-adjusted animal companion. This means your best bet on a purebred pup is the one who grows up in the breeder's home, smack in the middle of everything—kids, vacuum cleaners, doorbells, and pots and pans clattering in the kitchen. Steer clear of breeders who raise their dogs primarily in cages and the so-called "puppy mills" that crank out dozens of litters each year that may go straight from a cage on the farm to a cage in a store. Cage-reared puppies often don't get enough handling or exposure to new situations, and eating, sleeping, and excreting in the same small area goes against their instincts. The result can be a shy, fearful, or otherwise poorly socialized dog.

A puppy who is well socialized will play happily with other puppies but take equal pleasure in climbing into your lap for a pat and a cuddle. Once that happens, try turning the little guy over on his back and cradling him like a baby. If he fights you, you're looking at either one of the dominant puppies in the litter (the belly-up posture is a submission gesture) or one of the less trustful ones. If he doesn't mind being held this way, give him a tummy rub. If he's still not complaining, you're probably going to have more of a problem convincing him you should stop. The key is to look for the puppy who's interested in you, as well as the one you're interested in. And look more than once. Dogs can change their moods just like humans, so don't let first impressions force your decision; come back again once or twice (preferably at different times of the day), and see if the same puppies react the same way.

IS AN ADULT DOG FOR YOU?

Although puppies are a barrel of fun and cute as the dickens, remember the wise old saying, "Age before beauty." Just because an adult dog is no longer young doesn't mean he doesn't have a world of things to offer you. Folks sometimes have the mistaken notion if you don't raise a dog from scratch, you'll only have trouble. Nothing could be further from the truth. Sure, it may be easier in some ways for a tiny pup to bond with you, but there are definite advantages to the older dog. For one thing, they've settled down from puppyhood and might even have had some training already. If you've never had a puppy, you might not realize just how much energy he has. Keeping up with a puppy can be exhausting—and you can't turn him off or send him to his room to play if you've had a hard day.

Look for the same clues for health problems as with a puppy, and ask the source of the dog if your veterinarian can examine the dog before you adopt him. If you're adopting directly from the previous owner, ask to see the dog's health records so you can check on illnesses, vaccination history, and spaying or neutering (older dogs have probably already been "fixed," which is a bonus).

Far more so than with a puppy, an adult dog is a "what you see is what you get" proposition. Most all pups are cute, cuddly, and passive, but some will grow up and stay that way, and others will grow up to be the canine equivalent of Jesse James. An adult dog's personality is pretty much set, giving you a better handle on how well he'll fit into your household and whether or not he'll get along with any other pets. Since he's got all his adult teeth and is past the energetic phase of frantic puppy activity, a full-grown dog is less likely to do wholesale destruction and his longer attention span makes him easier to train.

If you have your heart set on a purebred, opting for an older dog may be easier than you think. There are a large number of breed rescue clubs that specialize in placing dogs of their particular breed who have been found as strays, taken from unsafe situations, or simply retired from the showring or the racetrack. Adopting a rescued stray, a retired show dog, or racing Greyhound will give you all the joys and benefits of dog ownership . . . and do a great favor for the dog, too. Check the classified ads in newspapers under the breed in which you are interested, contact breeders (they advertise in dog magazines), or call your local humane society for more details.

One last thought about the "secondhand" dog: A dog of any age can be trained and will adapt to—and be a loving, loyal companion for—a new family. You really can teach an old dog new tricks!

MAD ABOUT MUTTS: ADOPTING A MIXED-BREED DOG

They go by a dozen different names, and not all of them are complimentary. But whether you call them mutts, curb setters, or crossbreeds, there's one thing you can always count on about a mixed-breed dog: No two of them look alike! In fact, my pal Mary Jo says that's what she likes best about them. "It makes me feel special to know no one else has a dog quite like mine," she likes to say.

A mixed breed is just what it sounds like: a dog who doesn't come from a single purebred mother and father (of the same breed, that is). Sometimes mixed breeds are created by design, as with popular mixes like the Cockapoo (Cocker Spaniel and Poodle); Peekapoo (Pekinese and Poodle); and various retriever, German Shepherd, and poodle/terrier mixes. Otherwise, mixed breeds are just the result of nature taking its course.

Picking a mixed-breed puppy is a more of a roll of the dice than a purebred when it comes to size and instincts. You pretty much know how big your Beagle puppy will get, that he'll want to follow his nose constantly, and that he'll bay instead of bark. If you know the breeds of the mutt puppy's parents, you'll have a good idea what to expect. For instance, a Golden Retriever/German Shepherd mix will most likely be a good-size dog, with a potential weight range of 60 to 90 pounds and a fun-loving yet protective personality. Otherwise, you'll just have to be surprised. Some of the most special stories about dogs come from owners whose mixed-breed pups turned out to be something totally unexpected.

If you're not looking for a dog to show or work, or if you don't have your heart set on a particular breed, you can't go wrong with a mutt. Crossbreeds actually tend to have fewer of the health problems that may pop up in some of their purebred counterparts. What's more, the animal shelters are overflowing with mixed-breed dogs. Most purebreds can count on finding a home, but when you adopt a mixed-breed dog, you're giving him a new lease on life.

PEDIGREED PLEASURES: ADOPTING A PUREBRED DOG

Purebred means a dog whose ancestry can be traced back for generations through dogs with similar characteristics. The term "pedigreed" usually means a purebred dog has the paperwork to prove his breeding. Organizations like the American Kennel Club (AKC) run a registry

TALES FROM THE COUNTRY VET: MUTTS HAPPEN

I think the question I dread the most from a new client is, "What kind of dog is he, Doc?" Sometimes the dog looks so much like a particular breed I can get away with saying, "Well, he's a Labrador retriever mix of some kind." Other times, it's just not possible to tell.

Even a dog's looks won't tell you the whole story—it's easy to be fooled. Remember, we are the ones who decided a certain look, body shape, coat length, and so on add up to a particular breed. To a dog, none of that matters—it's just another dog.

Case in point was a dog my cousins had when I was young. His name was Duffy, and he looked for all intents and purposes like an Old English Sheepdog. Some fanciers of the breed even asked my aunt one time if she ever showed him. Well, it turns out Duffy was a mutt after all. He "happened" at a dog show, where the owner of a Standard Poodle and the owner of a Standard Collie got a little careless. The Collie's flat coat relaxed the Poodle's curls just enough to create a big, shaggy dog—a breed my cousins promptly dubbed the American Oops.

of purebred dogs. If an AKC-registered male Pomeranian mates with an AKC-registered female Pomeranian, then the entire litter can be registered as purebred Pomeranians.

You might be interested in a purebred because you want a dog of a certain size or temperament, or you might have a hankering to hunt him or show him. Purebred dogs come in a variety of coat types, each of which with its own appeal. If you enjoy spending a lot of time with a dog and giving him hands-on attention, you'll probably take pleasure in a dog whose coat requires regular brushing or styling, such as the Golden Retriever, Maltese, or Poodle. On the other hand, if you want to spend active time with your dog, you may prefer one with a short, easy-care coat. Buying a purebred dog offers you the opportunity to acquire a dog who has been bred not only for a specific look but also for health and temperament. Quite often the parents and sometimes even the grandparents of the dog can be examined for good health and compatible personalities.

A MATTER OF BREEDING

You name the job, and dogs have probably been bred for it. Dogs have been specifically bred for dozens of tasks over thousands of years. We developed breeds to help us hunt, herd or guard our flocks, protect our property and family, haul heavy loads, pull sleds or carts, and even do pest control duty. We even bred them tiny to be foot warmers and flea catchers. But no matter what the dog's original purpose, people soon learned a dog's number one skill is being man's best friend.

Today, it's a rare dog who fulfills his heritage as a worker, but all those generations of breeding for specific instincts still have a powerful effect on the dog's behavior. When you decide to bring a dog into your home, it's important to consider whether his instincts will match your lifestyle. For example, the Jack Russel Terrier is a cute little pooch who keeps turning up in films, TV shows, and commercials. He's a friendly and spunky little dog, but he's a terrier, a "ground dog." Terriers were bred to dig out burrows and even go down them after critters like rabbits and foxes. If you have a prize garden, a terrier is bound to give it an unwanted relandscaping. As long as they're breathing, they'll be digging, too. Doing a little bit of homework on the original purpose of a breed will help you figure out if it fits with your home and lifestyle—and help avoid an unhappy ending.

When you begin the quest to find just the right dog, ask yourself the following questions:

- What size dog do you want, and is this size compatible with your living quarters?

- How much time can you spend exercising/training/playing with a dog?

- What types of activities will you enjoy with your dog? Is your lifestyle active or sedentary?

- How much can you afford to budget for a good brand of dog food?

- Do you have a yard or access to a nearby park where your dog can play?

- How much time and effort can you devote to grooming your dog?

Once you've answered these questions, it's time to begin researching compatible breeds. Check your local library for books and articles about the breeds that interest you, and talk to people who are knowledgeable about them: other pet owners, breeders, and veterinarians. Thoroughly investigate breed characteristics. If you have a computer and online access, search the internet for web sites and breed interest groups.

WHICH BREED IS RIGHT FOR YOU?

The American Kennel Club divides dogs into seven groups: Sporting, Working, Terrier, Toy, Hound, Herding, and Non-Sporting. These divisions give you a rough idea of which breeds to consider first. For instance, if you enjoy hiking, jogging, or watersports, one of the Sporting dogs is likely to suit you best. These include such well-known breeds as Labrador and Golden Retrievers, Irish Setters, English

Springer Spaniels, Cocker Spaniels, and Brittanies, as well as the lesser-known American and Irish Water Spaniels, English and Gordon Setters, the various pointing breeds, and English Cocker Spaniels.

If your motivation for acquiring a dog includes protection as well as companionship, consider a Working breed such as the Doberman Pinscher, Boxer, or Standard Schnauzer. Although they tend to have gentle personalities, the size alone of a Great Dane or Newfoundland is enough to lend a feeling of security. These breeds also enjoy participating in various dog sports, such as sled dog racing for Alaskan Malamutes, Siberian Huskies, and Samoyeds, or carting for Rottweilers, Bernese Mountain Dogs, and Saint Bernards. While Working breeds can be formidable protectors and wonderful friends, they are probably also the most independent-minded. Good, humane, consistent—and preferably early—obedience training is particularly important for these pooches. They are also very large dogs, so if your grocery budget is limited, you may want to consider breeds that are smaller but just as protective, such as Terriers and Toys.

Terriers are well known as the farmer's best friend, keeping rats from the grain and foxes from the henhouse. These feisty dogs come in a variety of sizes, from the king-size Airedale to short-legged diggers like Cairn, Norfolk, and Norwich Terriers. The terrier propensity for barking and his protective attitude makes him a fine watchdog, but he can be a little overenthusiastic on this count, so proper training is important again. Since they come in a variety of sizes and coat types, there is a Terrier to suit just about any home.

When you think of a watchdog, a toy breed is probably the last one that leaps to mind, but size is not necessarily the only factor that qualifies a dog for this job. Toy breeds are alert, often the first to give the alarm when anyone approaches the house. Criminals admit it's a dog's bark, not his size, that deters them from breaking and entering. Of course, the company these dogs provide is also a benefit of owning one of them. Toy dogs have been bred as companions for at least 2,000 years, and they will happily take their place in any home, large or small, as long as it contains a lap in which they can cuddle. From the Pug, a Mastiff in miniature, to the elegant Toy Poodle, it's hard to go wrong with one of these diminutive dogs.

Like the Sporting breeds, Herding breeds are suited to families with an active lifestyle. Dogs who were bred to herd are intelligent, independent, and love having a job to do. Teach them a skill, such as rounding up the family for dinner or picking up dirty laundry, and you will soon wonder how you ever did without them. Popular herding breeds include Collies, German Shepherd Dogs, and Shetland Sheepdogs (Shelties). Because they are so smart, be aware you will need to begin training early to stay one step ahead of these dogs, but the results are well worth it.

> Whippets were bred to be racers. Known for their swiftness, they have a top speed of 37 miles per hour!

Hounds are the classics of dogdom. Among the oldest of dog types, they include the Greyhound, the Bloodhound, and the Beagle. Hounds are divided into two groups: sighthounds and scenthounds. Sighthounds are built for speed and give chase to fleet-footed prey such as hares and antelopes. Scenthounds tend to move more slowly, using their marvelously sensitive noses to track game. However, these defining characteristics are also the source of the major drawbacks to owning a hound. A sighthound is inclined to chase anything moving—and not stop until it stops or the dog drops. Scenthounds will likewise follow a trail to the ends of the earth. A good fence, long walks on a leash, and patient, consistent training are absolute musts. The reward for your investment is a dog with a sweet personality and variety in appearance, from the smooth grace of the Whippet to the thick-coated Nordic look of the Norwegian Elkhound.

Finally, there are the Non-Sporting breeds. These dogs don't quite fit in any other category. While they may once have served people by guarding coaches—like the Dalmatian—or retrieving downed waterfowl—like the Poodle—today they are bred strictly as companions. The Non-Sporting breeds come in a variety of sizes, coat types, and personalities, so from the laid-back Bulldog to the proud Lhasa Apso, this group contains something for everyone.

FINDING A BREEDER

Once you know you want a purebred puppy or dog and you have figured out the right breed for you and your home, the next step is to find a reputable breeder. Good breeders are committed to improving the breed. They are careful about breeding; have healthy, well-cared for dogs; belong to dog clubs or breeder organizations; and usually enter their dogs in shows. They try to eliminate health problems by screening their dogs for genetic disease. They keep current on information regarding vaccinations, canine medicine, and genetics.

To find a good breeder, ask your veterinarian or other dog owners for referrals. Breeders often advertise their dogs in such magazines as the *American Kennel Club Gazette, Dog Fancy,* and *Dogs USA,* all of which can be found nationwide. Attending a dog show is another good way to find breeders. Talk to breeders there, after they have shown their dogs (before competition, they will be too busy preparing the dog for the ring). Good breeders know their breed inside and out. They enjoy talking about their dogs, and they're willing to take the time to educate people who are new to the breed. Tell breeders the type of dog you're looking for—one who is quiet, active, friendly, easy to groom, good with kids, and so forth—so they can tell you if their breed

> There are 134 breeds currently recognized by the American Kennel Club.

THE TOP 10 DOG BREEDS

These were the most popular breeds registered by the American Kennel Club in 1996.

• Labrador Retriever (Sporting Group)

• Rottweiler (Working Group)

• German Shepherd Dog (Herding Group)

• Golden Retriever (Sporting Group)

• Beagle (Hound Group)

• Poodle (Toy and Non-Sporting Groups)

• Dachshund (Hound Group)

• Cocker Spaniel (Sporting Group)

• Yorkshire Terrier (Toy Group)

• Pomeranian (Toy Group)

suits your needs. Ask about a breed's personality and temperament. What are its grooming requirements? Does it have special dietary needs? Is it accustomed to children or other pets? What genetic problems affect the breed?

If you meet a breeder you like, make an appointment to see the dogs in their home setting. As you examine the dogs and facilities, talk to the breeder about standards and practices. An honest, responsible breeder will appreciate your concern and won't be offended by any of the following questions: How long have you been breeding dogs? How often do you breed your dogs? Why did you choose to breed these two dogs? Before you bred them, did you screen the dogs for health problems common to the breed? Can you show me the results of those tests? Do puppies come with a health guarantee or a veterinary health certificate? Do you belong to a breed club and subscribe to its code of ethics? Can your dogs perform the tasks for which they were bred (if it's pertinent to the breed in question)? Have your dogs earned any titles (conformation championship, obedience titles, tracking titles, herding titles)? Can you provide references from other buyers? What are the positives and negatives of owning this breed?

A good breeder will question you just as carefully. The questions she asks may seem personal, but her intentions are good: to ensure her puppies go to loving, lifelong homes.

A breeder may also require you to sign a contract agreeing to certain standards of care such as keeping the dog in a fenced yard or spaying or neutering a pet-quality dog. Some breeders withhold a puppy's registration papers until they receive proof the puppy has been altered. The breeder may also require you to return the dog if there ever comes a time when you can't keep it. In return for meeting such stringent requirements, you should expect to receive a healthy, well-socialized puppy at a fair price, as well as ongoing advice from the breeder regarding its care, grooming, and feeding.

Finding such a paragon of a breeder is not always easy. There is no canine version of the Better Business Bureau. Anyone can hang out a shingle proclaiming herself a dog breeder. As the buyer, it is your responsibility to screen the breeder carefully to ensure she follows reputable, responsible breeding practices. When you visit the breeder, take note of kennel size, exercise areas, cleanliness, state of repair, ventilation, lighting, and overall appearance. Are bedding and elimination areas clean? Is there an isolation area for sick dogs, show dogs, and newborns? Does the breeder feed a high-quality food, or are her animals raised on a generic diet? Is fresh water readily available? Does the breeder keep good records (including proof of vaccinations), store medications properly, and take steps to prevent worm infestation? In addition, rate the condition of the dogs and the socialization of the puppies. In the end, your own good judgment is what counts most.

CHOOSING A SHELTER DOG

When you adopt a dog from your local animal shelter or humane society—whether the dog you pick is a true "secondhand" pooch or a stray puppy—the odds are you'll not only be gaining a fine companion, you'll be saving his life in the bargain.

The same rules of preparation apply to the mixed breed adopted from the shelter as the purebreed purchased from the breeder. Sit down and figure out exactly what you want—and what you can handle—in a dog. That way, when you go to the shelter, the staff will be able to direct you to the dogs who fit your needs, and you won't be overwhelmed by too many numbers. Before you go to the shelter, it's a good idea to have a family meeting and make an actual list of the coat type, size, color, and so on, that you agree on. It's very easy to get sidetracked when a couple of dozen dogs are yipping and pawing at you through the bars of their cages.

Next, everybody in the household should pile into the car for the ride to the shelter. On the way, review how the selection process works. You should call your local shelters first for details on their specific procedures, but you can probably count on something like this: First, walk through the shelter to look at all the dogs and get an idea of who's available. Next, walk through again. Take your time. Have family members write down individually the one or two dogs they'd pick to adopt. Finally, walk through one last time, looking at all the dogs who were selected and comparing them to the list to see if they meet the criteria. If a dog doesn't match your needs, mark him off the list. Take your list of finalists and ask a shelter employee for more information about them.

Shelter employees see the dogs every day and should be able to tell you about a dog's personality and habits. If a dog was turned in by his owners, the shelter probably has more detailed information about his health and personality than about a dog found as a stray. Often, second-hand shelter dogs come with important background information: whether they get along with children or other animals, if they prefer men or women, and the type of home the dog was used to. Matching the dog's previous experience to your current situation can help a lot. For instance, some dogs may have a difficult time fitting into a home with very young children unless they came from a family with children. Look for the same health clues you would if you were buying a puppy: clear eyes, no coughing or sneezing, firm stools. Ask if the dog has been spayed or neutered, dewormed, and vaccinated.

Once you've heard what shelter personnel have to say, ask to meet the dog or dogs left on the list so you can make your choice. Don't forget, a dog in a shelter is away from its family, maybe for the first time. The loss of his home and the unfamiliar surroundings of the shelter are bound to affect the dog's behavior. Often, shelter enclosures are small, with little room for the dog to walk around. It's natural for a dog in this situation to be frightened, depressed, or withdrawn, so take these things into account when you make your decision.

Arrange to take the dog into a visiting room or to an outdoor area so you can get to know each other on a one-on-one basis. In this setting, the dog may loosen up, giving you a truer picture of his personality. Walk him around on leash. Does he pay attention when you switch directions? A dog who is willing and attentive is likely to be easier to train.

Whether you choose a puppy or an adult, look for a dog who is healthy and responsive. If the dog is friendly in a shelter environment, he's likely to be friendly in your home, too. But remember, a confined dog wants out, and even a somewhat shy pooch can be very solicitous when you walk past his cage. Take your time. Your decision is an important one.

HE FOLLOWED ME HOME: ADOPTING A STRAY

Sometimes, you don't choose a dog—he chooses you. Stray dogs seem to have a sixth sense about which homes will offer them a welcome. When a dog shows up on your doorstep, it may seem like fate, but take a deep breath and evaluate the situation just as you would if you were purchasing from a breeder or adopting from a shelter. Is your family ready for a dog? Is the dog right for you and your household? Do you have the time and resources to care for the dog? Is the dog healthy?

Approach a stray dog cautiously until you can be sure he's friendly and healthy. If he's wearing a collar and tags, you might be able to give his story a quick and happy ending by returning him to his family. (If you find he'll let you handle him safely, you can also check for registration tattoos, usually found inside the ear, on the inner thigh, or on the belly.) Unfortunately, most strays have no identification. You can put up signs and place ads, but you're going to have the dog in your home in the meantime, and many strays are never claimed. If you decide you are interested in giving the dog a home, your first step should be to take him to your veterinarian for a complete checkup and vaccinations. Only then should you bring the dog into your home, especially if you have other dogs who could catch any diseases or parasites the stray might have.

If you live out in the country, you're probably aware of the many dogs who are dumped off there by their owners in the hope they will find a place to stay.

Unfortunately, dogs are not capable of fending for themselves. If you can't keep a stray who comes to your door, the kindest thing to do is to take him to your local animal shelter, where he'll be fed and cared for until he can find a new home.

Bringing Fido Home

You've spent months thinking about getting a dog. You've done the research and found the dog who's just right for you. Now the day has finally come for you to take home the pooch of your dreams, but you may still not be quite ready yet. Before you bring your dog or puppy home, be sure you have the following supplies on hand:

Collar and tag. Order a tag engraved with your name and phone number several weeks before you bring your puppy home. Attach it to an adjustable buckle collar, and place the collar and tag on your puppy before you leave the breeder or shelter. As a puppy grows, check the collar frequently to make sure it isn't too tight. You should be able to slip two fingers between the collar and the puppy's neck. Collars can be made of leather or nylon, both of which are durable. However, puppies love to chew, and leather has an attractive scent and texture. If leather is your choice, wait until your puppy is past the teething stage.

If you have a puppy or are training your dog, you will need a training collar (also known as a choke collar). These collars are training devices to teach your dog not to pull as you walk him. These types of collars should only be used for training your dog; they are not substitutes for a regular collar. Also, never leave any kind of collar on a dog who's in his crate, unless you're there to supervise—it can snag and cause fatal choking. For the same reason, never leave a choke collar—whether nylon or metal—on an unsupervised dog.

Carrier. We're all familiar with the classic image of a dog riding with his head stuck out the car window, ears flapping in the breeze, and tongue hanging out; but a car in motion is not the place for a dog of any age to be roaming free. You'll need a crate (portable kennel) to safely contain your pooch during the ride to his new home as well as for future visits to the veterinarian and groomer.

Choose a sturdy carrier to hold your dog comfortably and keep it safe in case of an accident. Plastic airline carriers are lightweight, long lasting, and easy to clean. They are suitable for air travel if your dog will be living a globe-trotter lifestyle, and they can be secured in a car by running the seat belt through the handle. Wire crates are well ventilated and fold up flat when not in use. They can be covered to offer privacy or protection from the elements. Soft-sided carriers are comfortable and easy to transport. The zippered top and end closures make it easy to place the dog in and remove him from the carrier, and it's durable and easy to clean. On most airlines, soft-sided models are acceptable carriers for dogs traveling in the cabin, but they can't be used in the cargo area. Whichever style you choose, make sure latches are sturdy and edges are smooth, and be sure all screws, nuts, and latches are securely and properly fastened. Don't scrimp on quality to save a few bucks—it isn't worth risking your dog's life and safety.

Leash. Learning to walk on a leash is one of the first lessons of canine etiquette. Buy a lightweight, well-constructed leash. Leather leashes are handsome and durable, but skin oils can stain them and puppies delight in chewing on them. Nylon leashes are lightweight, colorful, and strong. Leashes made of chain are practically indestructible, but they are heavier than nylon or leather and can be noisy. A retractable leash gives your puppy the illusion of freedom but allows you to reel him in when necessary.

Food. A healthy dog needs the proper fuel. A dog's nutritional needs change over his lifetime—a puppy needs a different balance of nutrients than an adult or elderly dog—so talk to your veterinarian, breeder, or shelter for recommendations of the right food for your dog or puppy. Be sure you choose a food labeled as complete and balanced. Ideally, the label will state that the manufacturer has used feeding trials to substantiate the food's nutritional value.

Before you leave for home with your dog, find out the last time he ate, how frequently he's been fed, and what he's used to eating. If you plan to use a different food, introduce it gradually, over a two- to three-week period, by mixing the new food with the old food. An abrupt change in diet can cause diarrhea or vomiting.

Dishes. Food and water dishes come in a variety of materials. Each has advantages and disadvantages. Metal bowls are practical, last for years, and are easy to clean; but if you use canned food that has to be refrigerated, they can't be used to reheat a meal for your pup in the microwave. They're also fairly lightweight, making spills more likely. Ceramic dishes are decorative, can be personalized, and are generally both dishwasher and microwave safe. They're heavy, cutting down on spills and tipping, but they're also breakable. Some ceramic dishes made outside the United States contain high amounts of lead and shouldn't be used by people or animals. Plastic dishes are lightweight, colorful, inexpensive, and easy to clean and are also dishwasher and microwave safe. However, food odors can cling to plastic, and some dogs love to chew on them.

Grooming items. The basic items you need are a flea comb, a wire slicker brush, pin brush or rubber grooming mitt (depending on your dog's coat type), and a nail trimmer. A dog toothbrush and "doggie" toothpaste or cleaning solution are wise additions, too.

First-aid kit. You can buy a ready-made kit or put one together yourself. A complete first-aid kit should include a rectal thermometer, gauze bandages, scissors, bandaging tape, tweezers, antibiotic ointment, a needleless syringe for liquid medication, cotton swabs and cotton balls, hydrogen peroxide or syrup of ipecac to induce vomiting, and activated charcoal tablets to absorb poisons. Other useful items include a blanket and towel, a cold pack or a plastic bag to use as an ice pack, and rubber gloves. It's also a good idea to include your veterinarian's phone number, the phone number of the animal emergency hospital, and a first-aid handbook in the kit.

Toys. If you don't provide your dog with toys to help burn his boundless energy, he'll find some of his own—like your shoes, your tennis racquet, or even your portable radio. To channel his energy in the right direction, provide toys to exercise not only your pup's body but also his brain. A sturdy chew toy made of hard rubber will satisfy the urge to chew and soothe a puppy's aching mouth when new teeth are coming in. The noise from a squeaky toy is a surefire canine attention grabber—just be sure the noisemaker inside can't be detached and swallowed. A soft stuffed animal is the toy of choice for many dogs. Some curl up with it; others shake it and toss it in the air. Always choose a well-made stuffed toy, with no button eyes, bells, ribbons, or other attachments that could be easily chewed and swallowed. Finally, never give your dog anything as a toy resembling something you want him to leave alone—an old shoe, for instance. It's almost impossible for him to make the distinction between the shoe you want him to chew and the closet full of shoes you don't.

Bed. Your puppy will enjoy having a soft place to curl up and nap after playtime. From cushions to custom couches, paisley to plaid, there is an infinite variety of beds to suit not only each dog but also each decor. Choose a well-constructed, machine-washable bed. A wicker bed is classic, but remember, a puppy is a chewer and can easily destroy this kind of bed.

Choosing a Veterinarian

When you take your new dog home, he ought to be at the peak of health. A pup in this condition has no doubt been living in a healthful environment with good nutrition and all the right vaccinations against disease. Now, it's up to you to ensure he stays that way. You'll need to feed a high-quality food and offer balanced amounts of love and discipline, play, and rest. But perhaps most important of all, you will need to develop a close working relationship with your pup's veterinarian. When the two of you work as a team, confident in each other's abilities and observations, you maximize the quality of your dog's health care.

To find just the right veterinarian, ask pet-owning friends for recommendations. If you are new in town or don't know anyone who has a dog, don't worry. Most veterinarians belong to the American Veterinary Medical Association or the American Animal Hospital Association. You can contact one of these national organizations for a referral to a member veterinarian in your area. Once you get some recommendations, make an appointment for a first visit so the three of you can get to know each other.

This visit may include a brief physical exam so the vet can ascertain the pup's general state of health, but vaccinations should wait for another time. It's important for your dog's first impression of the clinic, doctors, and staff to be a good one. After all, everyone needs to trust their doctor—dogs included.

Communication is the foundation of a good client/veterinarian relationship. At this first visit, come prepared with the health records for your pup provided by the breeder, shelter, or previous owner and with any questions you may have about feeding, booster shots, flea and worm control, or anything else on your mind. Before you meet the veterinarian, you'll probably be asked to fill out a questionnaire with information about your dog's age, breed, sex, color or markings, and state of health. This medical history is the backbone of your pup's permanent record and will help the vet measure his growth and future health.

Don't be afraid to ask questions. And don't worry about "dumb" questions—if you don't know the answer already, it isn't a dumb question. For example, you might ask what food is best for a growing pup, how much and how often to feed, and when to switch to a diet for adult dogs. Use this time to evaluate your veterinarian's responses. Does she explain her answers fully, using terms that are easy to understand? Does she offer advice based on experience with other dogs of your pup's breed?

Consider, too, how comfortable the vet and dog are with each other. Some veterinarians have a better tableside manner than others. Ideally, your veterinarian will handle your pup with confidence and ease, holding him firmly yet gently and talking to him—and you—in a manner that is friendly and reassuring.

Every good relationship is also based on trust. In future visits, you should have no qualms about asking your veterinarian why she is recommending a certain course of treatment, medication, or lab test. The better informed you are, the better you will be able to follow through with the necessary care. Likewise, once you and your vet have talked it through, you should be able to feel absolutely confident this doctor will do her best for your dog.

When you leave the veterinarian's office after the initial visit, it should be with confidence that your pooch's health and well-being are in good hands: yours and your veterinarian's.

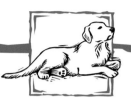

Understanding Your Dog

Dogs truly are humans' best friends. The strong bond between a dog and her owner is a natural result of the way a dog thinks. Even though there are hundreds of breeds of dogs and mixed breeds, they all have the same basic instincts and behaviors: the strong desire for companionship, the need to protect territory, and a complex way of communicating.

I've found that knowing the hows and whys of dog behavior helps me understand what makes dogs tick—and it makes me a better veterinarian. It'll help you, too, as you get to know your new friend. You just might be surprised by some of the things you learn about how puppies develop, the body language and sounds dogs use to get their point across, how dogs learn, and so on.

Communication

Just like us, dogs are social critters, living in communities called packs. It's one of the main reasons we get along so well. Our canine pals consider us members of their pack, and our home is their den. Social beasts that they are, dogs had to develop clear ways to communicate with each other—including vocal signals and a complex body language using face, ears, tail, and postures—so that every pack member could understand the message.

These very same communication cues are how dogs let us know what they're thinking. Whether it's a wag of the tail, a cock of the head, a bark, a whine, or a wiggle, your dog is making a clear statement—if you understand her language. Actually, it's fairly easy to learn "dog-ese." Just observe your pooch closely, and before you know it, you'll catch on to what she's trying to say.

Body Language for Beginners

Okay, we all know a wagging tail means a dog is friendly, right? Not necessarily. Dogs say lots of things with their tails—and not all of them are nice. A dog who is wagging her tail might be happy, interested, or confident, but she also may be scared, confused, or ready for a fight.

When you see a dog whose tail is wagging wide and fast, the message is almost always, "Glad to see you!" This is a happy, excited dog. On the other hand, a dog holding her tail loosely but horizontally wants to know a bit more about you. She might not be ready to welcome you with a big lick, but she's not going to challenge you either. The same is true of a dog whose tail is wagging slowly. She's still deciding whether you are a friend or foe. Watch out, though, for a dog whose tail is bristling or is held high and stiff, wagging fast. This dog is agitated and probably aggressive—and boy, does she mean business.

TALES FROM THE COUNTRY VET: MURPHY THE CLAIRVOYANT CANINE

Murphy was a "quad dog," one of those big old friendly mutts spawned on the quadrangle of a state university and picked up as a pup one spring by a soft-hearted biology major. The dog—a Lab/Shepherd/Golden mix of some considerable size—and the young man formed a quick and profound bond. They were inseparable, much to the displeasure of many of the fellow's professors.

The school year ended and the pair headed home for the summer. Being young and feeling his oats, the student was frequently out until all hours, particularly on the weekends. Yet, his parents always knew 15 minutes before he came home—Murphy would rouse herself from wherever she was sleeping, yawn loudly (waking the parents) and shake, and go lay down by the front door.

The entire household puzzled over the dog's apparent ESP. It didn't matter what time the student came home—Murphy always knew 15 minutes ahead of time! Until one hot night, that is, when her extrasensory gift failed her. But it was this failure that uncovered her secret: On the other nights, the windows were open and she could hear her master's car—badly in need of a muffler—as it exited the highway and turned down the quieter thoroughfares of her home neighborhood!

The position of a dog's tail tells a lot about her, too. A dog with her tail erect is confident and in control. The exact opposite is the dog with her tail tucked between her legs. Whether she's talking to you or to

Understanding Your Dog

another dog, the message is the same: "I give up!" Just because a dog's tail is down doesn't mean she's frightened, though. A relaxed dog may keep her tail lowered, although not between her legs.

Dogs communicate with both ends of their bodies. A cock of the head or twitch of the ears indicates interest or alertness but sometimes fear. When a dog hears or sees something new or exciting, her ears will go up or forward. Because the canine sense of hearing is so sharp, your dog often knows about the approach of a person or car long before you do. That's what makes her such a great alarm system. Her ears are built in such a way that they can be pointed in different directions, allowing the dog to quickly figure out where a sound is coming from.

Is a dog's head down and her ears back? She's scared or submissive. Sometimes, the fur along the neck and back of a frightened or submissive dog will bristle, too. Be especially careful approaching a dog in this mood. She might be timid or shy, but if she feels cornered, she's capable of launching an attack in self-defense.

A dog's pack instinct makes her a good observer who pays close attention to everybody and everything around her. You might not realize it, but your dog watches and listens to you all the time and learns your patterns of behavior. Sometimes it seems as if she can read your mind, but her ability to predict your every move is really just good observation skills at work.

Watch your dog's facial expression for more clues on how she's feeling. You might even catch her smiling—pulling the corners of her mouth back to show the teeth. Don't confuse this look with the snarl, a raised upper lip and bared teeth. A snarl is a definite threat gesture, but dogs probably smile for the same reason we do: to let folks—or other dogs—know they don't mean any harm.

Sometimes a dog uses her entire body to deliver her message. Rolling belly-up, exposing her neck and genitals, means "You're the boss!" An especially submissive dog may also urinate to express her deference to you or to another dog. The play bow is the classic canine invitation to fun and games: down on the front paws, rear end in the air, tail wagging. She may even paw the ground or bark in the attempt to lure you or another dog into play. The best response is to play bow back and then pull out her favorite toy or ball.

MAKING A JOYFUL NOISE

Body language is generally a silent method of communication (with the exception of the play bow), but dogs use their voices, too. They bark, whine, growl, and howl to get their point across. Barking is probably the most familiar sound dogs make. In the wild, only young wolves, coyotes, and foxes bark, but when dogs were domesticated, barking was one of the puppylike characteristics people liked and looked for when they were choosing which dogs to keep. Now dogs bark to say, "howdy," "pay attention to me," or to warn of trouble ahead. Some dogs bark when they're bored or lonely. Be careful how you respond to a dog's bark, or you might never get her to stop. Excited dogs love to bark, and if you yell at them to stop, they might just think you're barking back. You'll actually be teaching them barking is okay—just the opposite of the lesson you want them to learn!

One of the first sounds a young dog makes is a whine or a whimper to get her mother's attention. Mom feeds or comforts her when she whines, and soon the puppy learns people respond to that sound, too—especially when she wants to eat dinner or go for a walk. Dogs may also whine if they're frightened by loud noises, such as thunderstorms or fireworks.

Whining is cute when a puppy does it, but sometimes it gets to be too much. If your dog's whining becomes annoying, remember what you learned about how to stop barking. Instead of petting or comforting a

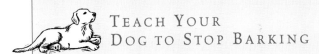

TEACH YOUR
DOG TO STOP BARKING

There are as many reasons for a dog to bark as there are things for her to bark at. To correct unwanted barking, first you have to find out why she's barking. For some dogs, barking is triggered by the doorbell, a passing car, or other common sound. Often this behavior can go on for quite awhile. Try a simple little homemade device called a shake can to curb your dog's barking. It's safe for the dog, easy to make, and often works like a charm.

Take an empty aluminum soda can, put a few pennies inside, and tape the top shut. When unwanted or excessive barking happens, toss the shake can in the direction of—not at—the dog. Do not try to hit her with it. The sudden loud rattling noise is often enough to surprise her into silence. This is your cue to jump in and tell her what a good dog she is now. Try to work it so the shake can appears to come out of nowhere. This way, your dog will connect you with good things (praise) and the shake can with bad things (barking).

If your dog is barking for attention, you can handle the situation two ways. The first is to ignore her until she stops barking. Don't pet her or yell at her. When she finally stops, praise her for being quiet. The alternative is to give the dog more attention than she wanted. As soon as your dog starts barking, put a leash on her and take her through a routine of sits, downs, comes, and stays. Continue this for a couple of minutes, then just walk away. Your dog will soon learn the sound of silence gets her the attention she wants.

whining dog, ignore her until she's quiet. Then reward her silence with praise or petting.

A growl is probably the easiest canine sound to understand. A growling dog is giving notice that she's ready to attack if you don't back off. Growling is a serious sign of aggression that shouldn't be ignored or laughed off. Don't let your dog get away with growling at you or anyone else, such as your veterinarian or groomer. Call in a professional trainer or behaviorist to help you evaluate the situation and get things under control. To learn more about aggression and its prevention, see Chapter 9, "Common Behavioral Problems and Home Remedies."

Everyone is familiar with the universal image of a canine—wild or pet—howling at the moon. The howl communicates excitement, warning, loneliness, or desire. Hounds howl when they have cornered their prey. Lonely dogs howl just to see if anyone else is out there. Howling in dogs is also as contagious as yawning in humans: When one dog howls, any other dog within earshot is likely to join in.

What's in a Name?

One of the most important ways you communicate with your dog is through her name. When your dog hears her name, she should jump to attention, ready for good times—even if it's just mealtime. Choosing the right name is a special part of dog ownership, so consider your choices carefully. Here are some things to consider to get you on the right track.

Your dog's looks. Spot, Blaze, Tiny, or Blackie are all tried and true dog names. The upside is they're descriptive, making it easier to identify your dog if she gets lost. The downside is there are a lot of other dogs

Understanding Your Dog

with those names. You might want to be more creative so your dog stands out from the crowd. A tall, leggy dog with a brindle coat—a Greyhound, for instance—might be named Savanna or Tiger, after the flat grasslands of Africa that might have produced an animal with this striped coat pattern.

Your dog's heritage. Investigating breed history is a great way to find the perfect name. A Scottish breed, such as a West Highland White Terrier, Scottish Terrier, or Cairn Terrier, might be named Murray or Stuart. Safari is a suitable moniker for a Basenji, the barkless breed from Africa. Tundra is a favorite name for Northern breeds like Alaskan Malamutes and Samoyeds.

Your dog's breed. Beagles, Bloodhounds, and Basset Hounds will follow their noses to the ends of the earth. Sniffer is a good name for one of these dogs, as is Sherlock or Gypsy. Lots of terriers are named Digger, and it's easy to see why. These dogs were once bred to go after varmints that lived in underground dens, hence their tendency today to excavate their yards.

Your pup's special traits. Why did you get your pup? If the two of you will be hunting or fishing together, you might go with the name Pal or Amigo. Border Collies are said to be the smartest of all breeds, so consider giving yours a name to match her intellect: Einstein or Newton, for instance.

Your puppy's registered name. Breeders often give litters a theme or names beginning with the same letter. A litter with a country music theme might have pups named Nashville's Yoakam, Nashville's Dolly, Nashville's Reba, and Nashville's Waylon. Registered names may include the kennel name or the names of the sire and dam. Thus you might have Cloverhill's Indian Summer, Craigwood Higgins of Switch-bark, or Magnolia's Prince of Thieves. Although these names appear on the dog's registration papers, they obviously aren't good choices to use around the house. The breeder or owner gives the dog a nickname, or call name. Craigwood Higgins of Switchbark probably goes by Woody to his friends.

Your hobbies and special interests. If you're a sports fan, you have lots of great names to choose from, whether your game is golf, tennis, basketball, football, track and field, or hockey. You might name a fleet-footed Greyhound or Whippet Carl, Jesse, or FloJo. Naming a Boxer is almost too easy: How about Frazier, Ali, or Sugar Ray?

Your favorite books, movies, or television shows. Lots of dogs are named Lassie in honor of the Collie of literary, film, and television fame. But you don't have to name your pet after another dog in a movie or TV show. Pick the name of any one of your favorite characters for your dog.

Helpful hints. Avoid names that rhyme with the word no, such as Mo, Snow, or Beau. You don't want to confuse your pup when you're training her. Avoid long or difficult names. Worcestershire may look impressive, but by the time you get it out of your mouth, your dog's attention will have long since shifted elsewhere. Finally, make sure the name is one you won't be embarrassed to call out in front of the neighbors.

TRAINING FOR PUPPIES AND ADULT DOGS

Now that your dog has a name to answer to—and you have a basic understanding of how to communicate with her—you can start teaching her how to live in polite human society. The pup's mother and litter mates taught her basic social skills. Now, it's your turn to further her education with the fine points, including housetraining, household manners, basic obedience, travel etiquette, and even a few fun tricks. Classes begin the day you bring your puppy home. Forget that old wives' tale about not training dogs until they're six months old. By that time, it may be too late. A young puppy learns things—some that you want her to know and some that you don't—every minute of every day, so you don't have an instant to lose.

But before you jump into training, be sure you understand the best ways to teach your dog. Dogs aren't born knowing what we expect of them. There are a million wrong or bad behaviors you could correct, or you can take the easy—and most effective—way of enthusiastically reinforcing the behavior you want. Puppies are smart, and sometimes it's a struggle to keep one step ahead of them, but by using positive reinforcement techniques—as simple as praise and petting—combined with limited humane corrections when needed, you can have a more-or-less model canine citizen.

The number one rule of dog training is don't hit—ever! Not only is it unfair (and inhumane) as a correction, it can actually backfire on you—sometimes with tragic results. Dogs don't hit each other, so they don't understand what getting hit is supposed to mean. They just know it's a physical threat and may eventually respond with their own physical violence in what they see as self-defense. The second most important rule is timing is everything. Positive reinforcement or corrections must happen immediately—in fact, almost simultaneous with the behavior—or your dog won't make the connection with her actions. Your secret ingredients for a well-trained pup are really no mystery at all. The secret is good old-fashioned patience and consistency.

Everything your puppy does is an opportunity to teach her. Praise her when she eliminates outside; that's the only way she'll learn the outside is the proper place. Praise her when she chews on a toy; that's the only way she'll learn to chew on toys, not shoes. If you find her chewing on your shoe, don't yell at her. Take the shoe away and immediately replace it with an appropriate toy, then praise her for being such a good dog and chewing on the toy. Instead of trying to catch your puppy doing something wrong, make every effort to catch her doing something right. It doesn't take a puppy long to catch on that she gets attention from you for doing certain things and that you ignore her when she does other things. A dog will do anything for attention, so your goal is to teach her which actions are socially acceptable and rewarded with your attention and which ones get her ignored.

Too often, dog owners fall into the trap of thinking dogs know exactly what's expected of them. The fact is dogs don't know the rules of your household, but they're eager to learn. Imagine it from the dog's perspective: You've just been picked for a team for an exciting new sport; however, nobody explains the rules to you. Of course, you have one major advantage over your dog: You can ask for clarification. Dogs can't, so it's up to you to make sure you're communicating all the rules to her consistently and in a way she'll be sure to understand. So instead of tossing your puppy into a situation where she doesn't know the rules, create an environment in which she can't help but succeed.

HOUSETRAINING YOUR DOG

Puppies and babies have a lot in common: They both need around-the-clock care, they both have to be picked up after, and they both do better on a regular schedule. The advantage a puppy has over a baby is housetraining takes much less time—that is, if you do it right.

Chow time. An important part of housetraining a puppy (or adult dog, for that matter) is her feeding schedule. Since housetraining is revolved around controlling what's coming out of your dog, it makes sense to begin by regulating what goes into your dog and when. This is especially important in these days of working households.

When you first bring your dog home, she may be as young as seven to ten weeks old. A puppy grows quickly—even a medium-size dog will go from two-pound pup to twenty-pound adult in six to eight months—and needs to eat three meals a day to build that much more dog. Not surprisingly, then, her diet must provide twice the energy as an adult dog's. This means puppies should only be fed a high-quality

THE BENEFITS OF CRATE TRAINING

A crate is really an excellent investment. It's durable and versatile, serving as housetraining aid, a safe mode of transportation, a bed, and a place of refuge when Rover is worn out or overwhelmed—and it lasts a lifetime. Wherever the crate is—bedroom, car, hotel, showgrounds—it's a little piece of home. More important, for the dog who has been properly introduced to the crate, it's her home base—a portable den. You see, denning is an important instinct in dogs. They like nothing better than to curl up in a small, cozy spot where they can feel warm and safe. Canine etiquette also demands all elimination take place outside the den, which explains why the crate is often so indispensable in housetraining.

You might be uncomfortable with the notion of caging your dog at first, but to a pooch, the crate isn't a jail. It's a safe haven. It's a happy coincidence for you the crate is a reliable way to help a new puppy avoid dangerous or destructive mishaps like chewing electrical cords or urinating on your new rug. Until a puppy's housetraining and household manners are reliable, she should cheerfully be put in her "den" any time you can't provide close supervision. And that includes bedtime when she should be crated in a room where humans are also sleeping. (Note: Overnight is the only time a puppy should be crated for more than four hours at a time. Adult dogs can be crated for up to eight hours but no longer.) Remember, the crate is your dog's den, her safehouse, her private shelter from the storm. It should always be open, always be where she can find it, and never be used as a punishment.

food specially formulated for growing dogs and should get it as part of a consistent feeding and exercise schedule that fits the needs of the dog and your household.

It's not a good idea to free feed your dog, leaving food out all the time. Not only does this make housetraining nearly impossible, it can also make your dog fat. A chubby puppy may look cute, but she'll be more prone to skeletal problems as she grows, especially if she's one of the larger breeds. So ask your breeder or veterinarian how much food your pup should get per day and divide that amount into three daily servings. For instance, if your Chihuahua puppy needs one cup of food daily, give her three one-third cup meals.

Toilet training. Here's a model housetraining schedule for a new puppy, which also applies just as well to an older dog.

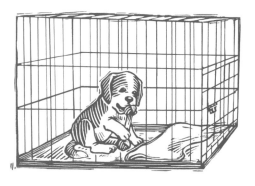

- At 6:00 A.M., take the puppy out of her crate and carry her outside immediately to eliminate. Bring her back inside, feed her one-third of her total food for the day, wait about 20 minutes, and then take her outside again. Praise her when she eliminates, and then head back inside for a little quality time. Put her in her crate so she can rest undisturbed while the family gets ready for work and school. The last person to leave the house should take her out to eliminate one more time.

The next time to take your puppy out should be around 12:00 P.M. A puppy doesn't really develop complete bladder control until around the age of six months, so it's absolutely necessary for a young dog to have her midday walk. This is a good time for the second meal, too. If you can't be home in the middle of the day, arrange to have a neighbor or pet sitter come in. Repeat the morning ritual: Take your dog outside from the crate, praise her for elimination, have some play time, give her a feeding, and then take another trip outside within 20 minutes of the meal.

- At dinnertime, when everyone in the household is usually home, repeat the noon routine. This can be a good time for a walk on leash, too. Let the dog hang out with the family during the evening, but be sure she's always under supervision. Remember, playing, eating, or drinking will stimulate the reflex to eliminate, so be sure to take the dog out after any of these activities. Take her out one more time before bed, then crate her in your bedroom.

Break the habit. Once you start shaping your dog's toilet habits, you'll need to focus on another important aspect of housetraining: teaching your pooch to respect your belongings. Once again, you want to create an environment that makes success easy and failure difficult.

First, use common sense: Put away anything you don't want the dog to chew on. Never give her your clothes or shoes to play with, unless you want your entire wardrobe to be fair game. Your dog can't distinguish between what's okay to use and what's off-limits.

Rotate her toys so she doesn't get bored with them. Put breakables where they can't get tumbled by accidental bumps or swept to the floor by the wagging tail of a rambunctious pooch. Always crate a puppy or confine her to a puppy-proof area like the kitchen or laundry room when you're not there to supervise.

Correct unwanted behaviors quickly, fairly, and briefly. Always positively reinforce appropriate behavior with praise and petting. In general, you should respond to unwanted behavior in one of three ways: ignore it, interrupt it, or redirect it.

Ignoring your dog is a social snub and lets her know the behavior isn't acceptable in polite circles. Give your dog the cold-shoulder treatment as part of an immediate correction for an unwanted behavior, but only keep it up for 10 to 15 minutes. (Any longer than that and your dog will have forgotten what happened.)

Interrupting the behavior helps break the habit and encourages the dog to try another strategy. Interruption works best when it comes unexpectedly; otherwise it can be programmed in as part of the cycle of unwanted behavior. For example, if your dog barks at the postman every day at 2:00 P.M. and your response is to go and get the shaker can, after a few days your dog will expect you to do it and just keep barking. The idea is to set up interruptions so the dog doesn't know it's coming. That way, the correction gets associated with the behavior and not with you.

Redirection is a more advanced technique and should be used once your dog has learned a basic vocabulary of commands such as sit, down, off, wait, leave it, and out. Once your pooch has these commands nailed down, you can use them to stop unwanted behavior in its tracks. So when your pup starts to jump up, you can tell her, "Sit!" or "Off!" instead. When she's eyeing your shoe as a chew toy, you can tell her to leave it (or if the shoe is already in her mouth, "Out!"). The wonderful thing about redirection—and an obedience-trained dog— is punishment is almost never necessary. You give the redirecting command, the dog responds, and you praise her. It's a win-win situation: The unwanted behavior stops, and Fido gets to be a good dog!

PUPPY KINDERGARTEN

Kindergarten for kids is a combination of structured teaching, informal learning, educational play, and free play—all of which give their rapidly developing minds an important head start in life. By the time first grade rolls around, they're already into the habit of going to school, and they have the basic skills for learning more complex concepts like reading and math. Puppy kindergarten works the same way: It gives young dogs a chance to get out of the house, meet other dogs and people, pick up some basic skills, and have a little fun along the way. The best time to enroll your puppy in class is after her vaccination series is complete, which should be at about four months of age.

Talk to your veterinarian, breeder, or local humane society about puppy kindergarten classes in your area, or ask friends or neighbors with well-trained dogs for their recommendations. As in any obedience training program, the first session of puppy kindergarten is usually held without dogs. This gives the trainer a chance to explain the methods to be used and answer any questions you might have. Expect the trainer to use positive methods, and avoid one who is harsh toward canine students.

Socialization is also an important part of puppy kindergarten. You'll play games like "Pass the Puppy," where everyone passes her dog to the next person. This teaches puppies to accept attention and handling from lots of different people, something your veterinarian and groomer will be grateful for! And always be sure to practice what you learn at home. Repetition is the key to learning in dogs.

BASIC OBEDIENCE FOR PUPPIES AND ADULT DOGS

After your puppy has graduated from kindergarten, the two of you can continue your education in a basic obedience training class. This is a must if you plan to compete in obedience trials but highly recommended even if you just want to reinforce what your puppy has already learned. After all, completing a single six-week class doesn't make your dog trained for life. Unless the two of you practice her skills at home on a regular basis—daily, at first—she'll lose them.

A basic obedience course should cover walking on a leash, sitting, lying down, and coming when called. The trainer may also include at-home care, such as brushing and nail trimming; practice exams to accustom the pups to having their mouths, ears, and feet handled; and advice on housetraining. It is also helpful to learn the psychology behind dog training, including timing, rewards, and corrections.

ON THE ROAD

A dog is one of the best traveling companions you can have. She doesn't whine about the length of the trip or insist on taking a short cut sending you 100 miles out of your way—and she's never a backseat driver. She is, however, a great listener who hangs on your every word and a powerful deterrent to people with less-than-honorable intentions. To ensure you and your dog make the most of your road time, teach your pooch early about the joys of car travel.

> Choose your classes wisely and carefully. In most places, there are no educational requirements for dog trainers so check credentials and get references.

Start off by taking her on brief errands, particularly ones that do not require you to get out of the car: the curbside drop-off box at the post office, drive-up bank teller, or the drive-through window at a fast-food restaurant. The bumps, turns, and sudden shifts of weight from a car ride are confusing to dogs, so keep your dog safe by keeping her in her crate or anchored to the seat belt with a specially designed pet harness. Running errands with your dog in the car is also a good way to teach her every car ride doesn't have to end up at the veterinarian, groomer, or boarding kennel.

To prepare for a long trip—longer than a half day or more—pack a separate bag for your dog. It should contain a supply of food; bottled water (or whatever water your dog is accustomed to drinking) to be

The Rules of the Road

When I make my farm rounds, my dog Toby always goes along for the ride. There's nothing she loves better than to go visiting, especially if it involves a ride in the car. But unless a pooch knows how to be a polite passenger, her presence can be annoying—and even downright dangerous. Teaching your dog manners for the car calls for the same approach as teaching her manners for the home: Positively reinforce acceptable behavior and correct unwanted behavior by ignoring, interrupting, or redirecting. If your dog really loves car rides, you can also use the old parents' dodge of "I'll turn this car around and go right home if you don't stop that," but be sure you actually do it. If nothing else seems to be settling your dog down, cut the trip short and bring her back home.

Teach your dog to wait until you give the okay before jumping into the car. This not only allows you to arrange your belongings—or the dog's—in the car, it also teaches your dog to respect your leadership, a must for compatible car travel.

As classic of a dog thing as it may be, don't let your pooch hang her head out the car window. The wind and dust can cause her eyes to become dry, and flying debris can cause serious—or even fatal—injury. Instead, your dog should ride in a sitting or lying position, inside the car, safely strapped in by her harness or riding inside her crate.

mixed with water along the way (to prevent stomach upset); dishes; bedding; a favorite toy or two; any necessary medication; heartworm preventative; and flea or tick products. Prepare a special spot in the car for your dog. If it's just the two of you, she may enjoy riding in the front seat. A large dog will probably be more comfortable stretched out in the backseat. Keep an eye on the sun's position in the car. It may be necessary to provide shade, especially if you're traveling through the hot Southwest or humid Midwest.

Stop every couple of hours so the two of you can stretch, take a potty break, and get a drink. Having a dog along is a good excuse to take a break and reduces the monotony of the drive, which can cause you to become sleepy or less alert.

Always snap the leash on your dog's collar and get a good grip on it before you open the car door. One glimpse of a passing rabbit or another dog at a rest stop, and Rover will be out of your control—and possibly into traffic—before you realize what's happening. Before you start your trip, always make sure your dog is wearing a collar and tags marked with your home address and phone number and with a number where you can be reached on the road. Special write-on tags are available for temporary use.

Two Easy Tricks

All work and no play makes Ginger a dull dog. Teaching her a few tricks brightens her day and gives her a job to do. The more a dog learns, the less likely she is to be bored—and boredom is a major cause of destructive behavior. To learn these tricks, your dog must already know the commands down and come.

Crawl across enemy lines. All the famous TV and movie dogs know this trick. They use it when they have to sneak up on the bad guys, get messages past enemy sentries, or heroically drag themselves back to their beloved masters, despite their injuries. The only props you need are some bite-size treats such as kibble, bits of hot dog, or cheese cubes. This trick will link a command your dog knows (come) with a new one (crawl).

To start, give your dog the down command. Once she's in position, back up a few feet and kneel down with a treat in your hand. As you call your dog saying, "Ginger, come—crawl," show her the treat and slowly pull it toward you along the ground. If Ginger stands up to get the treat, put her back in position and start over. If she crawls, even if it's only for a short distance, give her the treat and praise her. When she starts to get the hang of the trick, start making her crawl farther before you give her the treat.

Roll over, Ginger. Once your dog knows this trick, you can build on it to create more elaborate tricks, such as playing dead. As with the crawl trick, you need a supply of treats to teach your dog to roll over. Your dog will learn two new words for this trick: side and roll.

To start, your dog should be in the down position. Kneel in front of her with a treat in your hand. With an open palm moving in the direction you want your dog to lie (choose either left or right), encourage her to lie on her side. (If you want the dog to lie on her left side, use your right hand and vice versa.) As she moves into position, say, "Side." Practice this step several times until your dog has it down pat, rewarding her with a treat when she's successful.

The next step is to teach the dog to roll. With a treat in your hand, make a slow, complete circle as you say, "Roll." As your dog follows the motion of your hand, help her roll over, and give her the treat. Repeat this step until your dog can roll over without help. The roll should bring her back to the down position. When you are sure your dog knows the routine by heart, you can teach her to roll in the opposite direction.

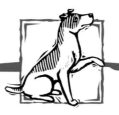

EATING RIGHT

Your dog is your best buddy, and you want to keep your buddy around for years to come. To keep your dog fit and happy, you need to make sure he's eating right. We've all heard the saying, "You are what you eat," and country folk know that's good advice to live by. Good, healthy food builds strong bones and muscles and keeps the body fit. The same is true for your dog. Don't think just any old food will do for your dog. Saving a few extra pennies at the grocery store may put money in your pocket for the short term, but in the long run, it's liable to cost you a lot in veterinary bills. A high-quality diet with just the right amounts of protein, fat, carbohydrates, vitamins, and minerals is a must for keeping your dog fit as a fiddle.

Your Dog's Basic Nutritional Needs

Anywhere people live, you'll find dogs. Our species has made its way into nearly every nook and cranny in the world, and we've bred dogs to go with us. One of the main reasons why dogs are so remarkably adaptable is their ability to survive on a variety of foods. While cats need nutrients only found in a meat-based diet, a dog's digestive system can pull the nutrients out of just about anything that's edible. That's why dogs don't need as much protein in their diets as cats. Still, dogs are naturally meat eaters, so meat protein is still an important part of a dog's diet. An all-around balanced diet is a six-part story: protein, carbohydrates, fat, vitamins, minerals, and water.

Water of Life

Fresh, clean water is more important to your dog than any other nutrient. About 70 percent of a dog's body is made up of water, which is vital for cell function and tissue lubrication. Dogs can live for many days without food, but a lack of water will kill them quickly. When it's hot outside, or if your dog is sick, especially if he is vomiting or has diarrhea, water is even more important.

If you drink bottled or filtered water because of the quality of tap water in your area, you may want to safeguard your dog's health by also giving him bottled water or investing in a good-quality water filter for your tap.

If you're taking your dog on a trip, don't leave home without either bottled water or a gallon or two of the water your dog is used to drinking. A change in drinking water can bring on an upset stomach. Mix your dog's regular water with the new water for a few days until his digestive system adjusts.

If your dog is suddenly drinking a lot more water than usual—and having to go out to urinate more often—it could be a warning sign of several serious health problems, including diabetes and kidney disease. Take your dog to the vet right away for a checkup.

BUYING DOG FOOD: WHICH IS BEST?

You've always suspected dogs eat better than people, and it may well be true. Pet food manufacturers spend millions of dollars researching the nutritional needs of dogs and cooking up tasty foods dogs like (and people will buy). Choosing a dog food that offers complete and balanced nutrition is the first step on the road to your dog's good health, but there are four other factors to consider as well: taste, digestibility, calorie level, and price.

Whatever food you buy should be labeled complete and balanced. This means the food has just the right amount of nutrients a dog needs to play hard and work hard. But how do you know a food is really okay for your dog to eat? Well, just like any other industry, pet-food makers have rules and regulations to follow. The Association of American Feed Control Officials tells pet-food makers the type of and amount of nutrients that should be in their foods. The manufacturers have to prove their foods meet these standards by conducting feeding trials or chemical analysis of their foods. Feeding trials are the best way to determine whether a diet truly meets a dog's nutritional needs. Look for the words "feeding tests," "AAFCO feeding test protocols," or "AAFCO feeding studies" to make sure the food was tested with feeding trials.

Companies that conduct feeding trials must certify they followed AAFCO guidelines and their nutrition claims are supported by test results. For information on foods certified as having met AAFCO's feeding trial requirements, call the Pet Food Institute's Nutrition Assurance Program at (800) 851-0769.

Taste test. Whether or not your dog likes the food is obviously important, too. You could buy the best food on the market, but if your dog won't eat it then its nutritional value isn't worth a hill of beans. However, just because a food tastes good doesn't mean it is good for your dog. (Think of the foods you love to eat that aren't good for you.) Read labels carefully to ensure the food your dog likes is also good for him.

Look out stomach. Digestibility means the amount of nutrients in a food that can actually be used by your dog's body. A food with poor digestibility often causes excessive gas, loose or large stools, and diarrhea. On the other hand, a highly digestible food provides the same level of nutrients in a smaller amount of food. This means less waste, resulting in smaller, firmer stools.

To determine digestibility, examine the label for high-quality sources of protein such as meat or poultry, cheese, and eggs. Labels don't contain digestibility information, but you can write or call the company for its figures. Look for foods with at least 75 to 80 percent dry-matter digestibility.

> About ten percent of the general canine population is subject to gastrointestinal problems that affect their ability to properly digest food, regardless of breed.

Counting calories. Growing puppies need food that is chock-full of calories and nutrients, but once they hit adulthood, this same diet will cause them to gain too much weight. Read labels carefully to see if a food is intended for puppies, adult dogs, or mature dogs. Some labels show the percentage of calories supplied by carbohydrates, fats, and proteins.

> To calculate how much it costs per day to feed your dog a certain brand, mark your calendar with the price of the food on the day you bought it. When you run out, divide the cost of the food by the number of days it lasted.

Money over matter. There's usually a direct relationship between a food's price and the quality of its ingredients. Like the saying goes, you get what you pay for. Although a premium food may have a high price tag, the high nutritional value it provides means you can feed less of it to your dog to meet his nutritional needs. You may even discover its cost per serving is comparable to generic foods. The good nutritional support this kind of food provides means your veterinary bills are also likely to be lower, providing an added savings.

There's an old saying among country folks: A man's most valuable possession is his reputation (well, that and a good hunting dog). The same is true for any business, and in particular, a company that makes pet food. So, the manufacturer's reputation is something else you should factor into the cost of food. A company that cares about its customers—canine and human—shows its concern by consistently producing a high-quality product, providing its address and phone number in easy-to-read lettering, and responding quickly and openly to questions about its food. It's easy to see how spending a little extra for a high-quality food can pay off in the long run.

READING THE LABEL

Ever try to read the ingredients on a package of dog food out loud? Some things are familiar enough, but eventually you run into some tongue-twisting 17-letter scientific words that only a research chemist understands. A good dog owner wants to know what's in his dog's food, but deciphering those labels can be pretty frustrating.

By law, manufacturers must label a food with a name, an ingredient list, a guaranteed analysis of the food's percentages of crude protein, crude fat, crude fiber and moisture, and the food's nutritional adequacy. Here's a quick guide to understanding what's on a label.

- Ingredients are listed by weight, in decreasing order. For instance, if the first ingredient is lamb, followed by rice, you know the food's main source of protein comes from lamb. But keep an eye out for an ingredient—wheat, for example—listed several different ways, such as flour, flakes, middlings, or bran. By splitting the general category of wheat up into these four different forms, each will appear farther down the list than if they were combined and listed as a single ingredient.

  Of course, even if you buy the same brand all the time, the ingredients may change from batch to batch. Manufacturers change ingredients depending on their price and availability, so check labels from time to time to see if the formula has changed. A change in the formulation isn't necessarily a nutritional problem, but changes in diet are sometimes the cause of digestive trouble in dogs.

- The guaranteed analysis panel will tell you if the nutrients in the food fall between the minimum and maximum percentages of nutrients, but not exact amounts. A particular brand of food may contain much less than the maximum stated on a label or much more than the minimum.

- A nutritional adequacy statement tells whether a food is meant for growth, maintenance, or weight loss; provides complete and balanced nutrition; and whether feeding trials or formulation was used to test the food's nutritional value.

Dry Food vs. Canned Food

Canned dog food looks more like something we'd eat than those chunks of dry kibble. Canned dog food looks more like chopped meat or beef stew, and dogs certainly love to eat it. But is canned food better for dogs than dry food? Not necessarily.

Studies show both canned food and dry food can be nutritionally complete. However, each has its own advantages and disadvantages. As long as the food meets your dog's nutritional needs, just weigh the benefits and potential problems against your dog's age and health, your budget, and your dog's preferences.

Dry foods help prevent the buildup of tartar and plaque on the teeth. Dry food can be left out all day without spoiling, and it is generally lower in fat and higher in carbohydrates than canned food. If your dog tends to gain weight easily, a dry food may be the best choice for him.

On the other hand, you might worry your dog will be bored with a diet consisting solely of dry food. Canned food is tasty, and most dogs love it. If you brush your dog's teeth regularly to remove plaque and tartar, a diet of canned food can be just fine. Of course, you can also mix dry and canned foods so your dog will have the best of both worlds.

Feeding Table Scraps: Yes or No?

I'll confess my dogs have had tastes of everything from pizza to barbecue. And I'm sure I'm not alone. Any dog owner who tells you he never slipped his pooch a piece of hot dog or gave him the leftover scrambled eggs is pulling your leg. There's nothing wrong with giving your dog an occasional small taste of people food—as long as it's really occasional. As a regular diet, it's not healthy at all. On the other hand, if really you enjoy cooking and would like to prepare your dog's food at home, here's a tasty recipe that will meet all his nutritional requirements.

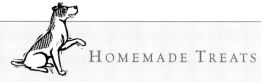

HOMEMADE TREATS

There's nothing like a homemade treat to satisfy your hungry pup. Here are a few easy recipes to try. (Note: Always make sure you check with your vet before giving your dog home-made snacks.)

Queenie's Favorite Dog Biscuits
- 4 cups whole wheat flour
- 1 cup cornmeal
- ¾ cup oil
- 1⅓ cup water

Preheat oven to 350 degrees Fahrenheit. Mix all ingredients together and roll mixture out on a floured board or table top. Cut with bone-shaped cookie cutter and bake on lightly greased cookie sheet. Bake for about 40 minutes. Let set until cool on a wire rack.

Doggie Diet Delight
- 1 whole (3 pound) chicken
- ½ cup honey
- 1 cup crispy rice cereal

Remove fat from chicken. Boil until the meat falls off the bones. Remove bones and grind meat. Add honey and mix well. Add crispy rice cereal and form into any shape desired, such as a large bone. Chill and serve.

(Recipes reprinted with permission from *Treasured Recipes* by Joan Dillon and Marlene Johnson.)

(Note: Check with your veterinarian before giving your dog any homemade meals. This is a basic diet for dogs with no known food allergies. Adjust the serving amount depending on your dog's appetite, activity level, energy needs, and weight gain or loss. Switch your dog to this diet gradually to prevent an upset stomach.)

Mix the following ingredients together in a big bowl:

1½ pounds ground meat (chicken, turkey, lamb), browned and drained of most of the fat	½ cup cooked oatmeal
	½ cup cooked barley, mashed
	½ cup grated raw carrots
	½ cup finely chopped raw green vegetables (broccoli, spinach, green beans)
1 medium potato, mashed and cooked	
2 cups cooked whole-grain brown rice	2 tablespoons olive oil
	2 tablespoons minced garlic

Store the homemade dog food in the refrigerator in a tightly sealed bowl, or divide it into daily servings and store it in the freezer, thawing a day or two at a time. You can keep the dog food up to seven days in the refrigerator.

Add the following when serving:

- Yogurt (a teaspoon for a toy dog, a tablespoon for a medium dog)
- A commercial dog multivitamin/mineral supplement
- Herbal supplement (depending on your dog's needs)

(Reprinted with permission from *The Consumer's Guide to Dog Food* by Liz Palika.)

YUMMY YOGURT

Dogs love yogurt, and it's good for them, too. If your dog has had to take an antibiotic, giving him plain, unflavored yogurt will repopulate his digestive system with healthy bacterial flora. (Make sure the yogurt contains an active culture.) Adding a small amount of yogurt to the food of a dog with gas can also cut down on his distress.

AVOID RAW FOODS

You'd think things like raw meat and eggs would be more "natural" for a dog's diet. After all, his cousins, the wolves and coyote, eat their food raw. But domestication has made our dogs' digestive systems a little more sensitive. Raw meat, poultry, and eggs may contain bacteria—such as salmonella—that can make your dog very sick, so it's best to always serve these foods cooked. In addition, raw egg whites interfere with the absorption of biotin, one of the B-vitamins. To prevent accidental illness from raw foods, keep a tight lid on the garbage, don't feed your dog tidbits of raw meat or poultry you're preparing, and forget about that fine old tradition of mixing a raw egg in a dog's food to help give his coat a healthy sheen. If you live on the Pacific Northwest coast, don't let your dog eat any fish he finds on the shore. A parasite common to salmon can cause potentially fatal disease.

Signs of salmonella or other bacterial poisoning in dogs are much the same as they are in people: loss of appetite, weight loss, lack of energy, fever, vomiting, and diarrhea. If your dog has any of these signs, take him to the vet immediately. Salmonella can be transmitted from dogs to people, so if your dog is infected, wash your hands carefully after handling him or anything he uses, such as food dishes or toys.

DEALING WITH THE FINICKY EATER

Finicky dogs aren't born, they're made. When you switch foods all the time because your dog turns up his nose at a certain brand or flavor or add a little of this and a little of that to make it taste better, you actually teach him that if he holds out, something more exotic will come along. Now keep in mind, a finicky eater is different than the dog who has been eating well and suddenly loses his appetite. If your dog normally enjoys his food but stops eating for more than a couple of

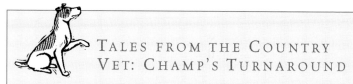

TALES FROM THE COUNTRY VET: CHAMP'S TURNAROUND

When a good friend asked me to watch his dog for a week, I was happy to do it. He started to give me a long list of instructions on the dog's proper care and feeding but broke off with a sheepish grin when I reminded him that I was the one who told him everything he knows about dogs.

The first day my friend was gone, I stopped in to see Champ—a fine-looking mixed breed—and give him his dinner. He was glad to see me, we had a nice walk and good play session, and I gave him a bowl of the high-quality dry kibble I'd bought for him. He didn't seem too interested in eating—not unusual for a dog whose human is out of town—so I just made sure he had enough water, picked up his food, said good-night, and went on my way.

By day three, Champ had gotten into the swing of the vacation schedule and sat expectantly in front of the cupboard where I'd stashed the bag of kibble, starting about 15 minutes before mealtimes. When my friend got home, a few days later, he called me frantically. "Champ is acting funny," he said. "What did you do to him?" "What do you mean?" I asked. "Well you know, he's a very picky eater. I have to open four or five different cans before I find the one he wants that day. But today he's just sitting in front of this cabinet, salivating like Pavlov's dog!" "Oops," I said, not really meaning it. "I guess since I didn't know Champ was so 'picky' I just fed him dry kibble. It looks like my ignorance was contagious, too, because now he doesn't know he's picky, either!"

days, get him into the veterinarian for a checkup. You may be convinced your dog will waste away to nothing if you can't coax him to eat, but if he's otherwise healthy, that just isn't so. Given no other choices, he'll eat whatever nutritionally complete food you give him—eventually. Here are two time-tested methods to conquer finickiness.

The "30 and out" method. Set down the dog's food and give him a half hour to eat it. At the end of 30 minutes, pick up the food, and don't feed him anything else until his next scheduled meal. Again, leave the food out for a half hour only. Most dogs are eating eagerly by the second day, although some may take three days. If your dog is single-minded enough to last till the fourth day without eating, you can try Plan B.

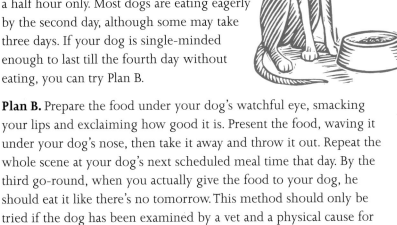

Plan B. Prepare the food under your dog's watchful eye, smacking your lips and exclaiming how good it is. Present the food, waving it under your dog's nose, then take it away and throw it out. Repeat the whole scene at your dog's next scheduled meal time that day. By the third go-round, when you actually give the food to your dog, he should eat it like there's no tomorrow. This method should only be tried if the dog has been examined by a vet and a physical cause for finickiness has been ruled out. This plan should not continue for more than one day.

A Salad Course? Why Dogs Like to Eat Plants

We usually think of dogs as being straight meat eaters—but they enjoy nibbling on grass and plants, too. There's no real scientific explanation for it, but there are a couple of educated guesses. Some researchers think the greens may provide certain vitamins or minerals missing in meat. Others point out that wild canines like the wolf and coyote hunt plant-eating animals and eat their entire prey—including their grass-filled stomach.

If your dog is one of those who enjoys a salad once in a while, don't deny him the pleasure. Just make sure the grass he's munching hasn't been treated with pesticides or fertilizer, and keep poisonous plants out of reach. Consider providing your dog with his own private planter of grass. That way, you don't have to worry about pesticides or worm eggs making him sick. Simply place some soil in a container, sow it with grass, oat, or wheat seed; water it; and watch it grow. Start a second container so it will be ready when your dog nibbles all the grass from the first one.

OBESITY

We all know that carrying extra weight isn't healthy for humans, contributing to such health problems as heart disease and diabetes, and the same goes for dogs. Obesity is the most common canine nutritional disease in this country, occurring in up to 25 percent of the population. Chubby dogs are more likely to develop serious diseases like diabetes, joint problems, infections, skin disease, and even certain cancers.

Of course, the best thing for your dog is not to let him get fat in the first place. Keeping dogs fit and trim works the same way as with people. Limit the intake of food to just enough to maintain normal body weight (in other words, follow label feeding instructions), don't leave food out all day for your dog to nibble, cut

Eating Right

out snacks, and be sure he gets enough exercise. Good habits start young, so if you have a puppy, don't overfeed him, and make sure the exercise he gets is the right kind: Too much jumping and running can be harmful to the bone development of a growing puppy.

To determine whether your dog is already too heavy, stand over him and check for a waist—a visible indentation behind his ribs. Then give him a hands-on test. Can you feel his ribs? They shouldn't be sticking out, but you should be able to find them through a layer of skin and muscle. If all you feel is rolls of fat, it's time to work with your veterinarian to develop a diet and exercise plan.

A veterinary checkup will ensure your dog doesn't have any health problems that would preclude regular exercise and a change in food and current exercise. Your vet will also advise you on the safest rate of weight loss; losing too much weight too fast can be dangerous. Monitor your dog's progress with weekly weigh-ins, either at the veterinarian's office or at home.

Since an overweight dog is also out of shape, start his exercise program slowly. Begin with short walks and work up to longer ones. Once your dog has lost some weight and built up his stamina, you can intersperse periods of jogging or running. Of course, use common sense when you exercise your dog. Go out early in the morning or evening, when it's cool, and stop long before your dog shows signs of exhaustion, such as panting or reluctance to continue. Your natural cooling system is better than your dog's (you can sweat; he can't), which means you can exert heavily for longer periods without overheating. Each year, many dogs die while gallantly trying to keep up with their humans on a long run.

To keep his diet on the right track, offer food only at mealtimes. If you can't resist giving treats, offer pieces of fruit (apples or bananas) or vegetables (carrots or broccoli). They're low in calories, and dogs love them.

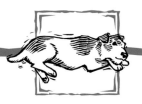

GROOMING HEAD TO TAIL

Even if you're too young to remember product slogans like, "Look Sharp, Feel Sharp, Be Sharp," you probably know good personal hygiene keeps you happier and healthier. Heck, if you've ever gone on a weekend camping trip, you know what I'm talking about. As nice as it is to get away from it all, there's something even nicer about getting back to a hot shower and shampoo. Well, the same goes for your dog: Clean, well-groomed fur, trimmed nails, clear eyes, and clean teeth keep her feeling more comfortable and looking and—let's face it—smelling better. To keep your dog at her best, you'll need to know some basic grooming skills—and when it's time to see a professional groomer.

Tools and Tips for At-Home Grooming

Coat care. Without regular brushing and combing, your dog's hair can develop mats. Matted hair pulls and inflames your dog's sensitive skin and can be even more painful to remove. Even dogs with short, flat coats need regular grooming to distribute skin oils and remove dead hair. With this in mind, every dog owner needs to have some basic grooming tools on hand.

A fine-toothed metal flea comb will last your dog's lifetime. Also use the flea comb to remove loose dead hair. If your dog's coat is heavily tangled, don't use a comb on it; you'll just end up hurting her.

Regular brushing keeps skin healthy by stimulating blood flow and distributing natural oils. If your dog has a short coat, a weekly brushing will usually do. But a breed with a thick, long, or shaggy coat, such as an Afghan or Old English Sheepdog, may require daily care. A wire slicker brush helps prevent mats from forming, and a curry brush or rubber grooming mitt removes loose hair quickly and easily. For best results, be sure you brush all the way down to the skin.

Use a natural bristle brush on shorthaired dogs. This type of brush can also be used on dogs such as Huskies and Collies who have "double coats"—a soft undercoat and weather-resistant outercoat. A steel pin brush is best for dogs with long coats, such as Maltese, Shih Tzus, and Yorkshire Terriers. Some dogs—Poodles, Bichons Frises, Kerry Blue Terriers—have curly or wavy coats requiring the use of a fine curved-wire slicker brush. For dogs with straight, flat, silky, feathered coats—like Setters or Spaniels—the pin brush or wire slicker brush is a good choice. Ask the breeder if your dog's coat requires a special type of comb or brush, especially if you plan to show the dog.

Before you begin brushing, mist your dog's coat with a spray-on conditioner. This helps the brush move smoothly through the fur, and cuts down on static electricity and broken hair.

To remove mats, work some baby oil or liquid tangle remover into each one. After several minutes, try to loosen and separate the mats, using your fingers or the end tooth of a comb. Carefully brush out the loosened sections, going slowly so you don't hurt your dog. In severe cases, the entire coat may need to be clipped.

> All dogs shed, but double-coated breeds, such as the Alaskan Malamute, Chow Chow, German Shepherd, Samoyed, and Shetland Sheepdog, shed heavily in the spring.

You may notice your dog's skin and hair are drier than usual in the wintertime, and her coat is crackling with static electricity every time you pet or brush her. Everyone in the house will feel better if you run a humidifier during heating season. After bathing, treat your pooch's skin with a conditioner made especially for dogs. A light coating of petroleum jelly can also help soothe dry or cracked footpads.

Pedicure. Don't overlook routine foot care. Because your dog spends so much time on her feet—without the protection of shoes—she's prone to punctures or wounds from glass and other sharp objects, as well as scrapes and abrasions from cement and gravel walkways. Examine your dog's feet on a regular basis to make sure she hasn't picked up any foxtails or goathead stickers. If grass seeds become embedded in the paw, remove them with tweezers. Clean small cuts, and apply antibiotic ointment or cream. Seek veterinary treatment for more severe cuts.

Small cuts or mild skin disease may cause infections in the sweat glands in your dog's feet, resulting in swelling or abscesses between the toes—a problem especially common in Bull Terriers, Dobermans, and Pekingese. Soaking the afflicted foot in warm salt water often will relieve the pain. A more severe or persistent infection calls for veterinary care, antibiotics, and other follow-up treatment.

If your dog steps in something gooey, soften it up by rubbing the foot with margarine, peanut butter, or shortening; then work it off. Apply ice to chewing gum to make it brittle and easier to remove. You can also try soaking the foot in a mixture of warm salt water and olive or mineral oil.

For dogs who live in regions with ice and snow in the winter, road salt and sidewalk ice-melt products can irritate the footpads. Washing and drying Muffy's feet after being outside helps reduce this painful condition, and it prevents her from swallowing the salt when she licks her sore pads. Booties are another option, although some owners— and some dogs—find them undignified. Dogs who spend time out in the ice and snow can also form ice balls between their toes. These can be prevented by using a silicon spray on the dog's feet before she heads outdoors.

Trimming a dog's nails takes equal measures of practice and perseverance. Keeping your pup's nails properly clipped means less wear and tear on your carpet and floors and less chance of a painful snagged, broken, or ingrown nail. The sooner you start getting your dog used to having her nails clipped, the easier it will be in the long run (especially if you get your dog as a puppy). Use nail trimmers made especially for a dog's nails. For best results, wait until your pooch is relaxed or sleepy. Clip just where the nail curves, beyond the point of the sensitive, pink area referred to as the quick. It's easy to avoid the quick if your dog's nails are clear, but dogs with dark nails require more precision. If you clip too much of the nail and hit the quick, use a styptic stick or styptic powder to stop the bleeding. (You can find styptic powder at pet shops or a veterinarian's office.) Or keep a bar of soap handy when you're trimming your dog's nails. If you nick the quick, just rub the nail along the bar of soap to stop the bleeding. A dampened tea bag is also good for this purpose. Trim your dog's nails about every two weeks, or as necessary. Nails need to be trimmed if they touch the floor when the dog is standing on a hard surface or if they make clicking sounds when she walks.

Dental care. Although dogs don't usually get cavities, they are prone to gum disease caused by tartar buildup. Tartar is a by-product of plaque, which is a soft, gummy residue left on teeth after eating. When plaque hardens, it forms tartar (or calculus), which in turn can cause the gums to get red, inflamed, and sore. This condition is called gingivitis. Gum disease is one of the most common problems veterinarians see in dogs. Besides causing bad breath, if periodontal disease gets bad enough, it can interfere with a dog's ability to chew and even effect internal organs, causing bacterial infections in the kidneys and heart.

Good dental hygiene can't start too young. If you begin tooth care in puppyhood, you can greatly reduce the chance of your dog developing periodontal disease. To brush a dog's teeth, use a small, soft toothbrush or finger brush with toothpaste or tooth-cleaning solution formulated for pets. (Human toothpaste foams too much, and the additives can upset your dog's stomach.) You can also wrap gauze around your finger and gently scrub the teeth with doggie toothpaste. To make toothpaste for your dog at home, mix baking soda (sodium bicarbonate) with a little salt and water. Apply it with a toothbrush or with gauze wrapped around your finger. Don't use this recipe if your dog is on a sodium-restricted diet.

Ideally, you should brush your dog's teeth every day, but even a weekly brushing will help. Tartar buildup has to be removed by your veterinarian, with the dog under anesthesia, so the extra effort of regular brushing will save you and your dog much more effort and expense later on.

Ears. Your dog's ears are delicate, sensitive, finely tuned instruments allowing her to pick up sounds far out of the range of human hearing. Considering how picky people get about their stereo equipment, you'd think everyone would understand how very important it is to take good care of a dog's high-quality "sound system." Infections or foreign bodies can seriously damage these marvelous creations, but just taking a few minutes each week to examine and clean your dog's ears will help keep them safe and sound.

The outer ear (also called the earflap or pinna) is most vulnerable to injury and infection since it's constantly exposed to foreign objects and dirt. Keeping the outer ear clean is the first line of defense against ear problems. Begin by examining your dog's ears daily. Healthy ears are light pink inside, with no apparent bad smell or discharge. Next, check for foreign objects. If your dog spends a lot of time outside, especially in tall grasses or wooded areas, she can get foxtails or ticks in her ears. Remove foreign bodies carefully with your fingers, then clean the ear with mineral oil. (Never use soap and water to clean a dog's ears; soapy water can cause an ear infection.) If a foreign body is deeply embedded in the ear or you're not confident about taking it out, have your veterinarian remove it. The old folk method of removing ticks—burning them with a blown-out match—is not really very effective. The best way to remove ticks is to grasp one firmly at skin level with tweezers and pull it straight out with a gentle, steady pressure.

Give your dog's ears a complete cleaning weekly or monthly, as needed. (Floppy ears usually need more attention than pricked ears.) Moisten a cotton ball or cloth with mineral oil, olive oil, or witch hazel, and gently wipe the inside of the ears. Don't use a cotton swab; it's easy to accidentally damage the delicate mechanisms of the inner ear. Certain breeds, such as Terriers and Poodles, have hair growing inside the ear that must be plucked to prevent wax and dirt from collecting. Ask a groomer or breeder to show you how to pluck the hair.

Always be on the lookout for the early warning signs of an ear infection, which is a not-so-uncommon problem for dogs. If your dog constantly shakes her head, has sore or red ears, or if the ears smell bad or have a discharge, take her to the veterinarian. Most infections of this type are caused by lack of air circulation and occur most commonly in breeds with floppy or furry ears. The moist, warm, dark environment is the perfect place for bacteria and yeast to flourish. By catching the early signs, you'll be getting your dog's developing ear infection under control sooner, preventing more serious complications that can lead to hearing loss.

Some areas of the country have regular problems with biting flies. A dog's ears are the perfect target for these annoying little critters, and repeated bites can result in fly-bite dermatitis, which leaves the ears scabbed and prone to bleeding. To help keep your pooch itch-free, apply a pet-safe (not a human strength) insect repellent to your dog's ears before she goes outside.

If your dog shakes her head and paws at her ears frequently but has no other signs of an infection, she could be bugged by ear mites. These tiny, spiderlike creatures invade the ear canal and feed on skin debris. A telltale sign of ear mites is dark debris that looks a lot like coffee grounds. Ear mites are most common in puppies and young dogs, since they're easily spread and pups spend a lot of time on top of each other while playing and sleeping. If you've got other dogs or cats in your home and one of them turns up with ear mites, it's best to treat them all. Most of the safest and more effective remedies are available only through your veterinarian, so don't wait to make the call.

Of course, good old commonsense prevention is the most important thing you can do for your dog's good ear health. Keep the ears clean, dry, and free from foreign objects and substances. Put cotton balls in your dog's ears at bathtime (if she'll stand for it) to keep water out of the ear canal, and dry the ears thoroughly when the bath is over. Most dogs love swimming, so be sure Muffy's ears are clean and dry after taking a dip. When it comes to ear care, an ounce of prevention is truly worth a pound of cure.

Eyes. Like the ears, your dog's "windows to the world" are sensitive organs. Check your dog's eyes daily, and wipe away dried matter from the corners of the eyes using a moistened cotton ball. Examine the eyes for redness, tearing, or discharge. Eye problems that don't clear up within 24 hours should be treated by a veterinarian. Among the eye problems affecting dogs are excessive tearing (usually caused by allergies, infections, injuries, or irritation), conjunctivitis (inflammation of the membrane that lines the eyelid, the conjuctiva), and foreign objects in the eye.

Tearing is especially common in toy breeds such as Poodles. If your dog's eyes seem to be tearing excessively, have your veterinarian take a look at her and see if it's possible to determine what the problem is and how to treat it. In some dogs, however, tearing appears to have no underlying cause. For whatever reason, they just shed lots of tears.

Especially in dogs with white or light coats, even normal tearing can cause dark stains beneath your dog's eyes. To help keep these stains under control, wash the area under the eye frequently using warm water and a cotton ball. Be sure to carefully trim away stained hair. Do not use soap near a dog's eyes—soasp in the eye will cause a corneal ulcer.

An unusual amount of discharge in the corners of the eyes or a reddish or "meaty" appearance of the conjuntiva are signs of conjuctivitis. Conjunctivitis is especially common in dogs who ride in cars with their heads stuck out the window or who spend a lot of time outdoors in windy, dusty weather. In mild cases, conjunctivitis sometimes clears up on its own. If the problem persists, take your dog to the vet for treatment.

Dogs will paw at their eyes to clean them (although most dogs aren't nearly as fastidious as cats), but if you see your dog continually pawing at her eye or squinting, she may have a foreign body in her eye. Examine the eyes in a well-lit room so you don't miss anything. To get a good look, pull down on the lower lid and up on the upper lid. If only one eye appears to be affected, compare it to the other eye to see how they differ. If you can't find anything or if you can't remove the object, take your dog to the vet for treatment.

Bathing Your Dog

Dogs don't need to be bathed frequently—only when they get dirty or smelly—but it's a good idea to accustom your dog to the bathing process while she's still young and open to new experiences. If you introduce bathtime as a fun, comfortable activity, it will be easier to accomplish when Lady is grown up and weighs 125 pounds.

Once again, follow the Boy Scout motto: "Be Prepared." Have everything you need laid out within easy reach before you start the water: brush, cotton balls, shampoo, and towels. Also, place a rubber mat in the bottom of the sink or tub so your pup won't slip and slide. Then fill it with warm—not hot—water.

Now it's time to add the dog. Brush her thoroughly, from the skin out, to remove tangles and loose hair. Tangles and mats only get worse

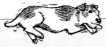

TALES FROM THE COUNTRY VET: DONDI MEETS THE REAL PÉPÉ LEPEW

Dondi was a dog who just never seemed to learn. Even after being sprayed twice by skunks, he couldn't stop himself from going after them again. The third time it happened, Dondi's owner called me in a panic. "What am I going to do?," she said. "He stinks for weeks, and I don't want to let him within half a mile, let alone in the house. Doctor, what can I do to get rid of this awful smell?," she exclaimed. I chuckled to myself, then gave her a few common household items to round up.

"Bathe Dondi—outdoors, of course—with his regular shampoo. Then rinse him with milk or tomato juice. Or try bathing him in a mixture of one quart of three-percent hydrogen peroxide, a quarter cup of baking soda, and one teaspoon of her regular shampoo. Whatever you use, be sure you rinse him thoroughly with water afterward."

"And that will do it?" Dondi's owner asked eagerly. "Probably not on the first try," I told her. You could just about hear her heart sink over the phone line. "Whatever method you use, you'll probably have to repeat it over several days before he smells like a dog again. But there's a plus side to this—I guarantee you'll appreciate how much more pleasant 'smelling like a dog' really is!"

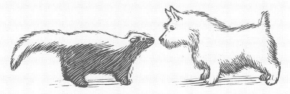

when they get wet, so make sure you remove all of them first. Place cotton balls snugly—but not deeply—in your dog's ears to keep out water and soap.

Next comes the fun part: Splashdown! (Make sure you're wearing clothes you don't mind getting wet.) Place your dog in the water, holding her gently but firmly. Wet her from the head down, making sure you keep water out of her eyes. Don't dunk the dog in water. Apply a shampoo specifically formulated for dogs. (Never use human shampoo—your dog's hair covers her entire body, not just her head, and the dose of ingredients she'll get from your shampoo may be too much for her.) Now, lather her up, working the shampoo down to the skin. If you're bathing a puppy with a flea-control shampoo, make sure it's safe for dogs her age. Always read and follow label directions carefully. Avoid getting the shampoo in your dog's eyes.

Keep talking to your dog during the bath, reassuring her and telling her what a good dog she is (even if she's trying to get out of the tub). Rinse her thoroughly, again using warm water. Be especially careful about getting shampoo in her eyes and ears when rinsing her head. Remove the dog from the tub, tell her what a good pup she is, and towel-dry her until she is damp. If it is hot and sunny, you can let the

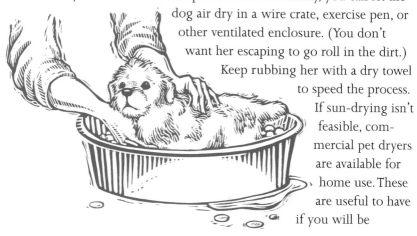

dog air dry in a wire crate, exercise pen, or other ventilated enclosure. (You don't want her escaping to go roll in the dirt.) Keep rubbing her with a dry towel to speed the process. If sun-drying isn't feasible, commercial pet dryers are available for home use. These are useful to have if you will be

Grooming Head to Tail

bathing your dog frequently or if your pup will grow up to be a very large dog. Otherwise, you can use a blow-dryer (if the dog is not scared of it) on a low, warm setting to finish drying her. Never use a blow-dryer set on hot or high, and avoid putting the blow-dryer too near her. Keep the dog in a warm, draft-free area until she is completely dry, especially if the weather is cold, damp, or windy.

To keep your dog clean and sweet-smelling after her bath, brush her regularly: weekly for a shorthaired dog and as often as daily for a dog with a long or heavy coat. Brushing removes dead hair, dirt, and parasites, and it distributes skin oils to keep Lady's coat shiny and beautiful. Plus, it just plain feels good. If you make bathing and brushing an enjoyable process—especially with a young puppy—it'll be a lot easier in the future.

The Professional Touch: When to See a Groomer

In today's busy world, a lot of us just don't have time to groom our dogs. Regular trips to a skilled, professional groomer are just the ticket for the busy dog owner. Some dogs are particularly high-maintenance, though, and it doesn't matter how much spare time you have—it may still be best to let an experienced groomer handle long, thick, or heavy coats. Other dog owners like to let the pros do the dirty work and keep their own interactions with their dog strictly for fun and learning. A professional groomer may also catch unusual spots, lumps, bumps, or even injuries on your dog you may have missed under all her hair.

A dog whose coat is heavily matted or soiled needs professional care. Removing mats is a time-consuming, delicate process, and mistakes can result in injury. In severe cases, some or all of the coat must be shaved. The professional touch is usually a must for show dogs, too. Grooming requirements for the showring are fairly strict (terrier coats must be plucked rather than shaved, for example), and an amateurish grooming job just won't put your dog in her best light.

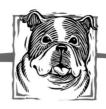

An Ounce of Prevention

"Dogs may be our best friends," says my old pal, Hoke Mitchell, "but I'm not so sure we're always theirs."

I don't like to make a habit of telling Hoke he's right about things, but he's got a point here. Dogs watch over our homes, keep us company when we're lonesome, warm our cold feet, and are generally at our beck and call. They'll positively knock themselves out just to be called "good dog." We've taken dogs into a world they were never meant to live in, full of strange diseases, speeding cars and trucks, food that comes out of a can or bag, and all kinds of things around our homes that seem good to eat but can sicken or kill a dog. Here's your ounce of prevention to help you do right by your best friend and keep him safe and happy.

MAKING YOUR HOUSE SAFE

A curious dog can get into every kind of danger a baby or toddler can—and some more besides. A dog's sensitive nose can sniff out intriguing—and potentially dangerous—off-limits items in hiding places a two-year-old child would never find.

Puppies are especially vulnerable because of their natural curiosity, lack of training and experience, small size, and still-developing bodies. Before your bring a puppy—or a dog, for that matter—home, look around your house and grounds with an eye for potential dangers: plants, pills, and poisons are the most typical. Make sure they're put away securely—well out of your dog's reach—and always put back where they were. A good place to start dog-proofing is with houseplants and yard plants. Many common plants are poisonous to dogs. To protect your pooch, you can remove poisonous plants from the premises, move them out of reach (in a hanging basket, for instance), put them behind a dog-proof barrier, or supervise the dog closely when he's around them.

POISONOUS PLANTS

We've already talked about how much dogs enjoy eating plants and grass. If you have a green thumb, you probably have lots of ornamental plants in and around the house. Since you grow them for show and never try to eat them, you might never have thought about whether they were poisonous. The leaves and stems of some plants contain substances that can be irritating and even toxic to the pet who chews on them. Common houseplants that can be harmful if swallowed include: dieffenbachia (or dumb cane), philodendron, caladium, and elephant's ear. Many yard plants such as flowers, shrubs, and trees are also dangerous to dogs. The bulbs of such flowers as amaryllis, daffodils, jonquils, narcissus, hyacinth, and iris are poisonous, as are azaleas, holly berries, hydrangea, ligustrum, privet hedges, oleander,

English ivy, jasmine, and wisteria. Of course, mushrooms and toadstools growing in the yard may be deadly. If your dog is the curious type, be extra careful about the kind of plants you keep around.

Next, search the house for pills or poisons that might be accessible to a puppy. Household staples such as aspirin, acetaminophen (Tylenol and similar products), ibuprofen (Advil and similar products), cold or cough medications, diet pills, and even chocolate can make your dog very sick or even kill him. Some household poisons are more obvious—snail bait, ant and rodent poisons, insecticides, and herbicides. Others—most notably cleansers and solvents—may not seem to pose a hazard but are attractive to dogs and extremely dangerous. There's still an annual death toll among dogs from antifreeze poisoning. The sweet odor and taste make puddles of spilled or discarded antifreeze a tempting—and poisonous—taste treat for animals.

The chocoholics among us would never think of the rich, dark stuff of our magnificent obsession to be anything but food of the gods. But the fact is, chocolate contains two compounds toxic to dogs: theobromine and caffeine. Baker's chocolate is among the purest—it hasn't been sweetened with sugar or mixed with other ingredients—and therefore the most dangerous. Just three ounces of baker's chocolate can kill a 20-pound dog. Although milk chocolate is less toxic by virtue of added ingredients, it's actually more dangerous because the milk and sugar make it more palatable. The bitter taste of baker's chocolate—or even semi-sweet chocolate—may discourage a dog from eating a fatal dose. You've heard the saying, "Life is like a box of chocolates. You never know what you'll get." Well, when a pooch bites into a box of chocolates, you know just exactly what he'll get: sick as a dog. Signs of chocolate poisoning include rapid heartbeat, muscle tremors, vomiting, and seizures. Without treatment, the dog can lapse into a coma and die. So keep anything chocolate out of paw's reach, especially at popular chocolate gift-giving times like Valentine's Day, Easter, Halloween, Christmas, or Hanukkah.

TALES FROM THE COUNTRY VET: ANTIFREEZE CAN PUT YOUR DOG ON ICE

I've got to hand it my client, Larry. He does the right thing. Last fall, he was winterizing his pickup truck and accidentally kicked over a jug of antifreeze. Larry ducked into the garage to get some rags to clean it all up and came back to find his trusty mutt, Rusty, lapping up the spill. He hauled Rusty into the house and called my emergency number. "Look at the label," I told him. "Does it say 'ethylene glycol' or 'propylene glycol'?" "Propylene," Larry said. "Is that good?"

"On two counts," I reassured him. "Good for your car this winter—and good for Rusty. You see, it used to be that most all antifreeze was ethylene glycol. The problem is, it smells and tastes enticingly sweet, but it's extremely toxic. As little as two ounces can poison an average-size dog, causing loss of coordination, excessive drinking and urination, and vomiting. Without immediate treatment, the dog can die in as little as two hours. And it's not only dogs or cats who were getting poisoned, little kids would drink it, too. So antifreeze manu-facturers started switching over to propylene glycol, a much less toxic choice. As long as Rusty doesn't show any symp-toms, he should be fine, but you were right to call me."

Larry heaved a sigh of relief. "Thanks, Doc," he said. "Any-thing else I should know? Any other advice?" "Sure," I said, wishing Larry could see my devilish grin. "Stick with that brand of antifreeze... and bring out the cleanup rags before you start to winterize your car next year."

While most dog owners can understand why any living creature, dog or human, would be attracted to chocolate, many make the tragic mistake of assuming their dogs won't be attracted to potentially dangerous substances that don't seem to be edible. Because dogs don't have hands, they use their mouths to investigate new things. The safest course of action is to put anything that isn't dog food or a dog toy safely out of reach. Poisons—including household cleaners, bleach, and the like—are best kept on high shelves or in cabinets secured with child safety locks.

Post your veterinarian's number by the phone, and keep a good pet first aid book on hand—one that includes a comprehensive list of common poisons and what to do if your dog swallows them. If you know what the dog ate, take the container with you to the veterinarian. If your puppy is vomiting but you don't know what he ate, take a sample of the vomitus to help the veterinarian make a diagnosis.

A DOG-SAFE YARD

Now that your yard is landscaped with dog-safe greenery, plants, and flowers, there are a few more touches you need to make it a complete home for your dog: a strong fence with a gate that latches properly and easy access to shade, shelter, and fresh water.

Whatever type of fencing you choose, make sure it's sturdy, with no way for your dog to escape. He shouldn't be able to jump over it, dig under it, or squeeze through a hole. If your pet is a confirmed digger, you may have to thwart him by lining the ground beneath the fence with concrete. Some homeowners like the open fields look and decide to put in one of those underground electronic "invisible" fence systems. If you're thinking of going that route, remember, although this type of fence might effectively keep your dog in, it won't keep other dogs or intruders out. Also, some dogs figure out—by trial and error or just by accident—if they run through the shock or ultrasonic burst that these systems count on to keep the dog on your property, there's nothing to stop them from heading into the next county. If you have the low-tech but reliable old-fashioned kind of fence, it's also not going to help much without a well-maintained gate. The gate should be hinged to close and latch automatically when you enter or leave the yard, with no way for Rover to nose it open.

Just as when you're looking for a home for yourself, finding where to place Rover's doghouse depends on three things: location, location, location. The ideal site is shaded during the summer and offers protection from the elements in the winter. If you live in a wet climate, place the doghouse in a high area with good drainage. Of course, a doghouse should have a floor so Rover doesn't have to sleep on the cold, damp ground, and raising the doghouse off the ground provides extra insulation. Some doghouses are designed with raised floors. You might want to surround the elevated area with boards or place hay underneath it so the wind won't whistle under the doghouse. For further protection from the wind, place the doghouse so the door faces south or east. As a general rule of thumb, most cold winds come from the north, northeast, or west.

If you plan on keeping your dog in a doghouse, don't keep him there for longer than eight or nine hours at a time—and even so, this should only be done if you are at work or will be away for the day. Also, check with your vet to determine the most comfortable outside temperature for your dog. What's adequate for one dog may be different for another, since a dog's comfort level will likely depend on his type, health, and age.

There's no doubt having a yard to let Rover out into is a marvelous convenience, especially on cold or rainy nights. However, you still need to make sure your dog has constant access to fresh water, and you still need to pick up after him every day. Things can pile up pretty quickly (no pun intended!), causing problems with odors, insects, parasites, and unpleasant encounters with Rover's paws, the lawnmower, or even your bare feet.

CHOOSING A DOGHOUSE

Back when I first started practicing veterinary medicine, most doghouses were rickety wooden structures, usually with a mournful old hound dog chained to them. If the dog was lucky, he might have a ratty scrap of old carpeting to lay on. But dogs today have it made. Modern prefabricated doghouses are designed for canine comfort and easy human maintenance.

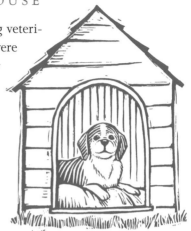

Even if your dog spends most of his time in your home, a doghouse gives him a place to hang out when he's in the yard and offers shelter from sun, rain, and snow. Of course, not just any old doghouse will do. Consider size, shape, design, and placement when you're buying. You don't have to give your dog a mansion, complete with air-conditioning, but you do owe your dog a comfortable, safe, clean, and inviting place to hang out when he's outdoors.

Your dog should be able to stand up, turn around, and lie down comfortably in his house. Don't assume bigger is better. A cozy doghouse retains heat, helping your dog stay warm in winter, and appeals to his denning instinct. If you are buying a doghouse for a puppy who will grow to be the size of a pony, buy it for how large he's going to be and provide plenty of bedding or block off part of the house until he grows into it.

Choose a house with a slanted or sloping roof so rain and snow won't accumulate and weigh it down. A removable or hinged roof makes it easier to clean the inside of the house. If the house has to be put together, it should be easy to assemble and disassemble, with sturdy latches that are easy to fasten and unfasten.

The doorway should be protected by a baffle or canvas flap to prevent rain and wind from blowing inside. An off-center entrance allows your dog to curl up in a corner away from cold winds. Make sure the doorway is high enough for Rover to walk in without having to stoop and the roof is high enough inside for him to stand with his head erect.

If you buy or build a wooden doghouse, be sure it's finished with a nontoxic paint—especially if your dog is a chewer. Wooden exteriors should be smooth so your dog doesn't get splinters in his paws or scrape his skin on the surface or on protruding nails. Sand down any rough or sharp edges. Like a wooden deck, a wooden doghouse should be treated with sealant to protect it from water damage.

Line the doghouse with a pad, a blanket, straw, or hay. A plastic mat or pad is durable and easy to clean. A blanket is soft and can be thrown into the washing machine as needed. Straw or hay is inexpensive and easily replaced, but it can be prickly or harbor insects.

Bedding in the doghouse must be cleaned or changed regularly. Wipe down plastic mats, and wash blankets or bed covers weekly in hot water to remove odors and kill parasites such as fleas and their eggs. Replace straw or hay regularly so it is always clean and sweet-smelling. During flea season, treat the bedding and the interior of the doghouse weekly or as directed on the label with a pyrethrin-based premise spray or powder. Remember: Once you acquire a shelter for your dog, keep it clean and well maintained for your dog's comfort.

> If you decide to build a doghouse yourself, consider using cedar wood. Cedar is popular because it has a pleasant scent and a reputation for repelling fleas.

PROPER IDENTIFICATION

One of the responsibilities of being a parent is making sure a child knows his address and telephone number. Parents patiently remind their children if they ever get lost, they need only find a police officer and tell the officer where they live. A good, permanent, and easily recognized ID—complete with your current address and phone number—is the best way to make sure the four-legged members of your family always find their way home safely, too.

There are three types of identification for dogs who fit this bill: tags, tattoos, and microchips. Each has its advantages and disadvantages, but no one method offers complete protection. Used together, however, they provide the best chance of a happy reunion with a lost dog.

ID tags. Most everybody knows to get a collar and tag for a dog. The classic canine ID tag is a simple and inexpensive way for your dog to carry your name and phone number. However, the collar-and-tags form of identification does have its drawbacks. The collar can come off or be removed deliberately by an unscrupulous person who finds the dog and wants to pass it off as an unidentified stray. Tags must also be updated when addresses or phone numbers change—something that often gets relegated to the "one of these days" list during the hustle and bustle of a move. (And, unfortunately, a move is a prime time for pets to get out and get lost.)
Tags with outdated information may be of just as little help as no tags at all. To top it all off, tags jingling on a collar can be annoyingly noisy, especially in the middle of the night.

Nevertheless, a collar and tag are the first line of defense against loss. Use a buckle-type flat or round collar with a sturdy D-ring for attaching tags. Never use a choke collar for anything except supervised training sessions. It's just too easy for it to snag on fences, shrubs, or other items and strangle an unsupervised dog.

Try to choose a distinctive collar and tag so it becomes part of your dog's unique description. For example, there are plenty of black Labrador retrievers in the world, but yours would stand out if he had a bone-shaped lime-green ID tag on a neon pink collar. The tag should be engraved and include your name and your day and evening phone numbers. These days, some experts advise against including the dog's name, since putting the dog's name where anyone can see it may make it easier to steal her. Leaving the dog's name off the tag can also help if someone finds your dog and tries to claim ownership. Certainly if you know the dog by name and the person claiming to be the owner doesn't, it makes it clear who's telling the truth.

There are options for an ID tag other than the classic metal tag, which may rust unless it's made of stainless steel. Plastic tags are sturdy and don't jingle as loudly as metal, but they can also fade and become brittle with age. A small metal or plastic identification barrel attached to the collar is a distinctive variation on the ID tag. These eye-catching devices unscrew to reveal a slip of paper on which you can record not only your name and phone number but important medical information about your dog, too. Engraved metal ID plates can be attached directly to flat collars, and some nylon collars can have your phone number woven or imprinted on them directly.

If you are moving or traveling with your dog, buy a temporary write-on tag with your new phone number or the phone number of a friend. Temporary tags are widely available through veterinarians, animal shelters, pet supply stores, and grooming shops. Ideally, however, you should provide your dog with an engraved ID tag listing not only your new address and phone number but also a contact name and number for your previous neighborhood. If your dog gets lost along the way, rescuers might not be able to reach you immediately at your new address. Some humane societies have a permanent ID tag registry system. The stainless-steel tag is engraved with the name of the humane society, the society's phone number, and a registration number. As long as you notify the humane society when your address or phone number changes, the tag will always be current, no matter where you go.

Tattoos. A tattoo is also a visible form of identification, but unlike a tag, it is permanent. Employees at research laboratories and animal shelters know to look for tattoos, and federal law does not permit laboratories to use tattooed dogs. A sticker or sign on your car, fence, or your dog's kennel noting your pet is tattooed can help ward off professional dog thieves.

Most tattoos are placed on a dog's belly or inner thigh. Tattoos remain the most legible when given after a dog reaches adult height. Avoid tattooing the inside of a dog's ear (as is done with racing Greyhounds); thieves have been known to cut off tattooed ears to prevent identification.

Tattooing can be done at a veterinary office, with the dog under anesthesia, or by a qualified individual at a dog club or other organization. The procedure is not painful, but it is noisy and time-consuming, so if your dog is squirmy or aggressive, he might require anesthesia.

Although a tattoo is a permanent identifying mark, it must be registered to be of any use. Otherwise, the finder has no way of contacting you. The registry can assign you a code to be tattooed on the dog, or you can use a number that will remain the same for your lifetime, such as a social security number (if you don't mind your personal information walking around in public). Phone numbers and birth dates are poor choices because they change frequently or can be shared by a large number of people.

The major disadvantage of a tattoo is not everyone knows how to contact a registry, or it may not be immediately clear which registry your dog is signed up with. However, tags and tattoos can be used in combination, with the dog wearing a tag bearing a registry phone number. As with the humane society permanent tag, it's crucial to let tattoo registries know if your address or phone number changes.

Microchip implants. These sound like something out of a science fiction movie, but many "chipped" dogs and cats have been reunited with their owners already through this rapidly growing means of reliable, permanent identification. The chip is typically placed under the skin at the scruff of the neck through a procedure much like giving a vaccination. It is virtually painless, and a single implantation lasts a lifetime.

Available only through veterinarians and animal shelters, microchips are tiny, battery-free devices, no bigger than a grain of rice. Each is programmed with a unique, unalterable code number and some sort of information identifying the chip's manufacturer. Microchip registries keep your personal information on file, listed by the chip's code number. Code numbers are also cross-referenced to the animal hospital or humane society that implanted the chip—an important backup in case you move and forget to forward your new address to the registry. Specially designed scanners read this information from the chip, through the dog's skin. Before implanting a chip, the veterinarian scans it to confirm the code, then scans again after implantation to make sure everything is working properly.

A microchip sends a signal only when it's activated by a scanning device. The scanner decodes the signal and displays the identification code on a liquid-crystal display window. Veterinary and humane organizations recommend microchipping as a safe and effective way of identifying lost pets and ensuring their return. This type of identification has the potential to save the lives of thousands of dogs who would otherwise die in shelters, unrecognized or unclaimed. As with tattoos, national registration is the best way to make sure you and your microchipped dog are reunited—as long as the registry has your current address and phone number.

REGISTERING YOUR DOG'S IDENTIFICATION

Listing your tattooed or microchipped dog with a national registry gives you access to the registry's database and services, which often include 24-hour notification, a tag with the registry's phone number, and an indication that the dog wearing it is tattooed or chipped. Often, registries also work through a network of animal shelters across the country. However, many shelters and laboratories now routinely scan strays they receive for microchips, and even if you haven't listed your dog with a registry, the lab or shelter can still find the owner of a chipped dog by tracing the code number to the veterinarian who implanted the chip.

Your dog is a beloved member of your family. Protect him from permanent loss by ensuring he is well identified. Should he ever escape from your watchful eye, you'll be glad you did.

NEUTERING AND SPAYING

It might seem strange to you to find this topic in a chapter on preventive care, but it might also surprise you to learn that spaying a female dog before her first heat and neutering a male before he reaches sexual maturity can prevent many health and behavior problems. Contrary to the old wives' tale, female dogs absolutely do not need to have one litter (or one heat) before being spayed. In fact, just the opposite is true. Spay and neuter surgeries are easy to perform on young puppies, taking less time and requiring less anesthesia thanks to new technology and new drugs. Young pups recover more quickly than older puppies or dogs, and the long-term health benefits include a much smaller risk of developing mammary tumors and no risk at all of dangerous uterine infections or testicular cancer. Dogs who are spayed or neutered before they hit puberty have a much greater chance of living a long, full life.

Another common myth about spaying and neutering is an altered dog will get fat. The truth is weight gain and loss in dogs runs by the same rules as for humans. Too much food and not enough exercise—not spaying and neutering—are what causes dogs to gain weight.

Spaying or neutering a dog also has a positive effect on behavior. If there's a female dog in heat practically anywhere in the known universe, an unaltered male dog will know it. He'll try to get out, roam far and wide, mark your furniture and other things with urine, and may become overly aggressive. An unspayed female goes through the discomfort and mess of heat (estrus) about twice a year, during which she may also try to escape or become more unpredictable in her behavior. Without the ebb and flow of those hormonal tides, spayed and neutered dogs are more consistent in their temperament—which makes training easier—yet their zeal in protecting you and your home is undiminished.

Neutering has one other important benefit that often gets overlooked: It prevents the birth of unwanted puppies. According to the Humane Society of the United States, 25 to 35 million dogs are put to sleep each year because there just aren't enough homes for them. Even if you let your dog have a litter and find homes for every last puppy, that simply means there's an equal number of puppies somewhere else who didn't get those homes and will end up being put to sleep. Your dog should be altered by the age of four to six months, unless your veterinarian recommends waiting longer. Spaying or neutering is a one-time investment (many animal shelters even have low-cost spay and neuter programs), dramatically lowering your dog's risk of several serious disease (including some cancers), and doubles your dog's life expectancy.

PREVENTIVE HEALTH CARE

Preventive pet medicine can catch problems before they become serious, saving time and money. How does preventive medicine work? It's a lot like caring for your car, really. You routinely check the oil and the air pressure in the tires and take the car in for regularly scheduled maintenance. By doing the same thing for your dog—examining him at home on a weekly basis and scheduling an annual veterinary exam and vaccinations—you can nip health problems in the bud and even extend your dog's life.

Regular veterinary visits. When you take your dog in each year for his veterinary exam, the vet doesn't just give him some vaccinations and send him on his way. He does a thorough exam: palpating the body to make sure all the internal organs feel normal and there are no worrisome lumps or bumps; checking the condition of the eyes and ears; listening to the heart and lungs; checking the weight; and taking the temperature. Because dogs age differently than people, this annual physical is comparable to you having a physical exam every five or six years. This is especially important if your dog is middle-aged or older because it gives the veterinarian a chance to find and treat health problems before they become serious.

Vaccinations. Most folks take it on faith that vaccinations are good for a dog and protect him against disease. They're right, of course. When puppies are born, they are protected by special antibodies produced in their mother's milk, but as they get older they lose this protection. That's why they need a series of vaccinations, usually starting at six to ten weeks of age, to stimulate their own immunity against disease. The vaccinations are repeated every three or four weeks until the pup is about four months old. Then he gets annual vaccinations to protect him throughout his life. These vaccinations protect your dog against such killers as rabies, parvovirus, and distemper and against other diseases such as viral hepatitis, leptospirosis, parainfluenza, coro-

VACCINATION SCHEDULE

During their first few months of life, puppies are vulnerable to disease, even with vaccinations, because the protection provided by the maternal antibodies has faded, and the vaccines have not yet had time to take effect. To protect your puppy during this time, be sure he comes in contact only with dogs and other puppies whose vaccinations are up to date. Of course, you want lots of people to play with your pup while he's young, but be sure they wash their hands first, preferably with an antibacterial soap. Here's the basic timetable for which shots a dog should get and at what ages.

• Parvovirus, 6 to 8 weeks

• Distemper/measles/parainfluenza, 6 to 8 weeks

• Distemper, hepatitis, leptospirosis, parainfluenza, parvovirus (DHLPP), 8 to 12 weeks

• Rabies, 12 weeks

• Coronavirus (optional), 12 weeks

• DHLPP, 16 weeks

• Coronavirus (optional), 16 weeks

• Parvovirus (optional), 18 to 20 weeks

• Rabies, 1 year, triannually thereafter

• DHLPP, annually after puppy series is completed

• Coronavirus (optional), annually after puppy series is completed

DOGS ARE THE BEST MEDICINE

Wouldn't it be great if doctors could invent an all-purpose wonder drug to relieve stress, promote weight loss, lower blood pressure, and help heart patients recover faster and survive longer? Well, they don't have to—it already exists. And it's not a drug... it's a dog.

Time after time, research shows what dog owners have always known: Sharing your life with a dog is good for you. The simple act of stroking a dog's soft fur reduces blood pressure and lowers stress levels. Cardiac patients who own dogs recover more quickly and have higher long-term survival rates. Dogs motivate us to get outside and walk, run, and play. The next thing you know, we're losing weight and looking good. That, of course, helps prevent us from getting heart disease in the first place. If the government really wanted to save money on health care costs, it would change the old slogan from, "A Chicken in Every Pot" to "A Dog in Every Home."

navirus, and kennel cough. If you live in an area where Lyme disease is common, especially if your dog spends a lot of time outdoors, the vet can vaccinate for that as well.

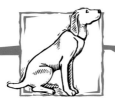

WHAT EVERY DOG OWNER SHOULD KNOW

"So, Doc. Should I bring Max in?" I must get 1,000 variations of that question every year. It's a good one to ask: Never assume a health problem will get better by itself. But you can save yourself a lot of time, money, and worry if you have a good working knowledge of the signs and symptoms of disease and injury. Once you can sort out what's a genuine (or potential) problem and what's not, you'll know when to wait and see—and when to get your "Max" to the vet.

Now remember, we don't award you a DVM at the end of this chapter, so don't try to second guess your vet. What you will be able to do is recognize the early warning signs so you know when to call the vet.

Early Warning Signs

I'm not sure where the phrase "dogging it"—putting out less than a full effort—comes from. Dogs work hard, especially when they're sick. A dog who's under the weather works hard to convince you she's just fine. That comes from thousands of years of instincts. In the wild, an obviously sick or weak animal (even a predator) is as good as dead. Even though she doesn't have to worry about that too much anymore, your dog's instincts still tell her to hide any signs of illness. You'll need a sharp eye and good observation skills to catch some of the more subtle clues. Of course, the better you know your dog, the easier it will be.

Some of the things to look for are basic: the way your dog looks, acts, eats, and drinks. For instance, she might look like she's gained weight, even though her appetite hasn't changed much, or like she's losing weight, even though she's eating more. A ten percent change in weight (which could be as little as a pound in a small dog) is something to bring to your vet's attention.

Usually, we know our dog is feeling good when she chows down on her food. It's not unheard of, though, for her to skip a meal or two, especially if it's hot outside. Any more than that is something to be concerned about. If your dog turns up her nose at food for more than two days, call your vet right away. Some diseases and medications cause dogs to develop eating habits that are downright out of the ordinary for them. A dog who has never been a food thief and suddenly starts raiding the garbage can or stealing food off the dinner table is telling you she needs a checkup or an adjustment of her medication.

A dog who starts drinking water like a fish could be developing diabetes or kidney disease. You may not be able to notice the dog's extra water consumption easily, but you should be able to pick up her increased intake by paying careful attention to what comes out the other end. She'll be producing much larger amounts of urine and have to go outside more often. She may also start having accidents in the house.

A healthy dog has a thick, shiny coat. A dull coat or one with rough, dry, or bald patches is a sign something's not right. The problem could be the type of food your dog is eating, a flea allergy, or another skin problem. Whatever the case, your vet's advice will help put your pooch back on the right track.

A more subtle sign of illness is what veterinary texts call "lethargy." (In simple terms, it means laziness or sluggishness.) A dog who's lethargic might show no interest in going for a walk, even though that's usually the highlight of her day. She doesn't want to play, not even her favorite game of fetch the tennis ball. Now, sometimes lethargy can be chalked up to a hot day, being sore after an extra long walk, or just feeling out of sorts. If it continues for more than two days, though, talk to your vet.

A familiar and not-so-subtle sign of illness is vomiting. Vomiting is not as dramatic a thing in the dog world as it is for us, and dogs may even vomit deliberately to get rid of something that doesn't agree with them (yesterday's garbage, for instance). Occasional mild vomiting usually isn't anything to worry about. But if your dog vomits frequently or several times in a row, has a fever, seems to be depressed or in pain, or has bloody or forceful vomit, you should call the vet immediately.

Taming a Turbulent Tummy: The "Quiet Diet" for Dogs

Sometimes, diarrhea is just the result of an upset tummy. Let your dog's digestive system rest by withholding food for a day. For the next two or three days, feed her bland meals of one part boiled hamburger meat or skinless, boneless chicken mixed with four parts rice, potatoes, or pasta. Your dog should also drink plenty of water if she has diarrhea. Entice her to drink by adding a little chicken broth to the water. If the diarrhea doesn't start to improve within a couple of days, take her to the vet.

The same bland diet can be used for mild vomiting. Again, withhold food for a day, then give a small amount of the meat mixture. If your dog keeps it down, you can give her a little more in a few hours. If this seems to solve the problem, feed a larger portion of the bland diet the next day, and return to her regular food the day after.

Finally, go on poop patrol. As unpleasant at it may sound, your dog's stool is a clue to her health. A healthy dog's stools are small, firm, and moist. Dry, hard stools that cause your dog to strain on elimination may be a sign your dog isn't getting enough water, or it may be a hint of another dietary or health problem. Squiggly, rice-shaped segments in the feces indicate worms. It's not unusual for an occasional stool to be loose or liquid or to contain mucous or even a tinge of blood. But diarrhea, straining, or mucous- or blood-tinged stool lasting more than two days should prompt a visit to the vet. If the elimination problem is accompanied by other signs—fever, vomiting, lethargy, loss of appetite, bloody diarrhea—call the vet immediately.

What Every Dog Owner Should Know

Giving a Home Exam

While a full-scale physical exam should be left to an expert (your veterinarian), your ability to perform a home exam is a valuable skill. It allows you to become familiar with your dog's entire body, so you notice instantly when something isn't right. Your dog's regular grooming session is a great time to perform a home exam. She'll enjoy the extra attention, and it's a good opportunity to spend some quality time together.

Skin and fleas. Start by looking for dry skin, dandruff, fleas, and flea dirt. To check for flea dirt, brush out your dog's coat over a white piece of paper or light-colored towel. If you see any little black specks, moisten them with a drop of water or smear them with a damp cotton ball. They'll turn red if they're flea dirt. Fleas, of course, can be picked up with a fine-toothed flea comb. Dip the flea comb in a bowl of soapy water—the soap holds them down and keeps them from jumping out, and the water drowns them. If you find signs of any of these problems, consult your veterinarian. She can advise you of the best products or treatments.

As you comb or brush your dog, pay attention to her reaction. Does she enjoy the feel of the brush going through her fur, or does she flinch when you touch a certain spot? Examine the area for lumps or sores. If you find an area that seems painful, make a note of its appearance. Is the lump hard or soft? Oozing or rough? Pass this information on to your veterinarian.

Eyes, ears, and mouth. The eyes should be bright and clear, with no redness or runny discharge. Tear stains beneath the eyes may indicate a problem. Besides looking into your dog's ears (they should be dry, with no discharge), sniff them, too. It sounds strange, but an unpleasant odor in her ear is a sign of an infection that may be out of sight in the ear canal. While cleaning your dog's teeth, take a look around her mouth. The gums should be a healthy pink, not pale or red.

Paws. Finally, examine your dog's paws. Do the nails need to be trimmed? Long nails can get snagged and break and are difficult to walk on. If they get too long, your dog can even become lame. Finish the exam with a soothing massage. It's a good way to deepen the bond between you and your dog.

Keep a written record of your home exams so you know what's normal for your dog. Note her eating, sleeping, and elimination habits, as well as activity levels. By referring to this health diary on a regular basis, you'll notice immediately if something has changed—and these records can be invaluable in helping your veterinarian diagnose any problems.

☎ WHEN TO CALL THE VET

Sometimes, the wait-and-see approach is best. Other times treatment just can't wait—your dog's life may hang in the balance. The important thing then is to stay calm, do what you can to control the situation, apply first aid as needed, and get her to a vet as quickly and safely as possible. There are times when a call to the vet—or a trip straight to the animal hospital—are a right-this-minute priority. Emergency situations include:

- Heavy bleeding, including any open wound or bleeding from nose, mouth, ears, or any other body opening.

- Difficulty breathing, swallowing, standing, or walking, including prolonged or frequent panting, staggering, or an uncoordinated gait.

What Every Dog Owner Should Know

- Fractures or dislocations. If you suspect a broken bone, don't try to find the break or set it yourself. Let a professional handle it.

- Loss of consciousness.

- Convulsion, electrocution, paralysis, shock, or persistent sneezing.

- Blunt trauma, including being hit by a car or getting caught in doors or machinery, even if there is no apparent serious injury. These kind of accidents may cause internal bleeding or injuries only a veterinary exam can detect.

If your dog shows any of these signs, don't wait to take her to the veterinarian. Waiting even for a few hours—and, in some cases, just a few minutes—can be fatal.

INFECTIOUS DISEASES

It's a different world of veterinary medicine than when I was a boy—and a better one, to be sure. The beloved dog of my childhood—a mutt I called Aspen—died of distemper. I still remember standing under the big oak tree in our yard, crying while my father dug in a small grave in the good, black earth. I promised myself when I grew up, I'd do my best so other kids wouldn't have to lose their dogs—and advances in science have kept me true to my word.

Fortunately, today we have vaccines to help prevent many of the killer dog diseases—and antibiotics to treat some diseases when they do strike. With the proper series of preventative vaccinations, your dog will most likely never suffer any of the diseases listed in this chapter, but I've described them just in case.

THE NOT-SO-MAGNIFICENT SEVEN

There are seven common and potentially fatal canine diseases you should protect your dog against with regular vaccinations: canine cough (also known as kennel cough), coronavirus, distemper, canine

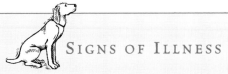

Signs of Illness

The following signs of illness can indicate potentially serious problems. If you notice any of these symptoms, you should call your veterinarian for a consultation:

- She seems tired or sluggish.

- She has trouble urinating or she's urinating more than usual.

- She's dragging or scooting her rear on the floor. She may have worms, her anal glands might be blocked, or she might have kidney disease or diabetes.

- She's drinking a lot more water than usual.

- She won't eat and misses more than two meals.

- She eats a lot but is losing weight.

- She's drooling a lot. She might have tooth or gum problems, or she could have gotten into something poisonous.

- Her gums are red or swollen.

- Her eyes are cloudy or red, she's squinting, or has a lot of discharge from her eye.

- She's gasping or short of breath.

- She flinches or whimpers when she's touched.

- She has any kind of lump on her body.

infectious hepatitis, leptospirosis, parvovirus (or "parvo" for short), and—the most dreaded of all—rabies.

Canine cough. This is a respiratory infection common to any situation where many dogs are kept together, such as kennels (giving rise to the

- She vomits, gags, sneezes, or coughs repeatedly.

- Her coat is rough or dull.

- She is unspayed and has a vaginal discharge.

- She coughs or vomits up blood.

The following signs of illness can indicate very serious problems. If you notice any of these symptoms, take your dog to the vet immediately:

- She's dehydrated. Pinch the skin at the back of her neck. If it doesn't return back in place quickly, she might be dehydrated. Another sign of dehydration is dry or tacky gums.

- Her gums are pale, white, or blue.

- She can not urinate.

- She faints or collapses.

- She has a seizure or convulsion.

- She becomes overheated.

- Her abdomen is enlarged. She might have a gastric torsion (a twist in her stomach), mammary tumor, heart or liver disease, peritonitis (inflammation of the abdominal lining), or pyometra (uterine infection).

- She's unable to use her back legs.

name "kennel cough"), animal shelters, and pet stores. The infection causes the trachea, larynx (voice box), and bronchi (the little branching tubes in the lungs) to become inflamed. Succumbing to the bacteria *Bordetella bronchiseptica*, an infected dog will develop a mild to severe cough, sometimes with a runny nose, five to ten days after exposure. It can be treated with antibiotics and plenty of rest, which is very important. As with all the Not-So-Magnificent Seven, prevention is the most sensible and humane choice. If you plan to board your dog or will be exposing her to many other dogs, be sure she's protected against Bordetella. The "double whammy" is often a good strategy: a liquid vaccine administered through the dog's nose combined with an injection for canine parainfluenza virus.

Coronavirus. A usually mild disease, coronavirus is spread when a dog comes in contact with the stool or other excretions of infected dogs. Although it rarely kills dogs, coronavirus can be especially hard on puppies or dogs who are stressed or not in the best of health. Suspect coronavirus if your dog is depressed, doesn't want to eat, vomits—especially if it's bloody—and has a bad case of diarrhea. Exceptionally strong-smelling stools, particularly if bloody or with a strange yellow-orange color, are also signs. If coronavirus is diagnosed, the veterinarian will give your dog plenty of fluids to replace those lost from the vomiting and diarrhea, as well as medication to help keep the vomiting and diarrhea to a minimum. A coronavirus vaccination is usually recommended if your dog will be meeting lots of other dogs—or their excrement—at parks, dog shows, kennels, and other boarding facilities.

Distemper. Around the world, more dogs die from distemper than any other infectious disease. This highly contagious virus is spread by direct contact or through the air. A hale and hearty dog can survive distemper, usually with relatively mild symptoms. On the other hand, if your dog's immune system doesn't come out fighting, her whole body can be overwhelmed by the virus, as well as bacteria that jump in to cause secondary infections.

Distemper usually happens in two stages. Three to fifteen days after exposure to the virus, the dog develops a fever, doesn't want to eat, has no energy, and her eyes and nose become runny. As time passes, the discharge from her eyes and nose starts to get thick, yellow, and gooey—the classic sign of distemper. If you haven't taken your dog to the vet before this symptom appears, you should take her now. Other first-stage signs of distemper are a dry cough, diarrhea, and pus blisters on the stomach. The second stage of distemper is even more serious, because the disease can begin to affect the brain and even the spinal cord. A dog in this stage might slobber frequently, shake her head, or act as if she has a bad taste in her mouth. Sometimes she has seizures, causing her to circle, fall down, and kick her feet in the air. Afterward, she seems confused, wandering around and shying away from people. Unfortunately, when the disease gets this far, there's not much hope for the dog to survive. Dogs who do survive often have permanent neurological (brain and nerve) damage. Distemper can also spread to the lungs, causing pneumonia, conjunctivitis, and inflamed nasal passages (rhinitis); it can also spread to the skin, causing it to thicken, especially on the foot-

> Distemper generally affects dogs under 12 months old.

pads. This form of distemper is called hardpad disease. Distemper is most likely to strike dogs as puppies between nine to twelve weeks old, especially if they come from an environment with several other dogs (animal shelter, pet store, breeding kennel). If your dog is diagnosed with distemper, your veterinarian will give her intravenous fluids to replace those she's lost, medications to help control the diarrhea and vomiting, and antibiotics to combat secondary infections.

Canine infectious hepatitis. This is a viral disease spread by direct contact. Mild cases last only one or two days, with the dog running a mild fever and having a low white-blood-cell count. Very young puppies—two to six weeks old—can suffer a form of the disease that comes on quickly. They have a fever, their tonsils are swollen, and their tummies ache. Very quickly they can go into shock and die. Onset is

BLOOD TRANSFUSIONS IN DOGS

When I first started practicing veterinary medicine, blood transfusions for cats and dogs were rare. But that's changed. In fact, in just the last 10 years or so, the technology of transfusion medicine for pets has grown dramatically.

Like people, dogs have different blood types. In general, a dog with a particular type of blood needs to get the same type of blood in a transfusion. Again, as in humans, there is one canine blood type that is a "universal donor"—it can be safely given to a dog of any blood type without ill effects. (While human blood types are coded A, B, or O, dog blood types are named by specific protein sites on the surface of their red blood cells.) Ideally, a dog should get her own blood type—but in a pinch, the universal donor blood will work.

The most common reason for transfusion is an accident—being hit by a car or suffering a serious wound in which a lot of blood is lost. Treatment of autoimmune disease (where the disease-fighting antibodies in the blood turn their attack on the dog's own body) or certain kinds of cancer may call for transfusions to replace diseased blood cells. Even some cancer treatments like chemotherapy may suppress production of certain blood cells (or destroy healthy cells), which must be replaced by transfusion. Transfusion can also be a lifesaver for puppies who have severe anemia from hookworm, internal bleeding from rodent poisons containing warfarin or similar compounds that produce hemorrhage, and diseases like canine hepatitis (a liver disease) and Willebrand's disease (similar to hemophilia).

quick and unexpected: The pup may be fine one day and in shock the next. The most common form of canine infectious hepatitis occurs in puppies when they are six to ten weeks old. They show the usual signs of fever, lack of energy, and enlarged tonsils and lymph nodes. A dog whose immune system responds well will start to recover in four to seven days. In severe cases, however, the virus attacks the walls of the blood vessels and the dog starts bleeding from the mouth, nose, rectum, and urinary tract. If your puppy has canine infectious hepatitis, she will need intravenous fluids, antibiotics, and maybe even a blood transfusion.

Leptospirosis. This bacterial disease is caused by a spirochete, which is a type of bacteria with a slender spiral form. The leptospirosis spirochete is passed in the urine of infected animals and enters a dog's body through an open wound in the skin or when she eats or drinks something contaminated by infectious urine. The signs of leptospirosis are not pretty. Early symptoms include fever, depression, lethargy, and loss of appetite. Usually, leptospirosis attacks the kidneys, so an infected dog may walk all hunched up because her kidneys hurt. As the infection advances, ulcers appear in her mouth and on her tongue, and her tongue has a thick brown coating. It hurts to eat because her mouth is full of sores and might even be bleeding. Her stools have blood in them, and she's very thirsty, so she drinks a lot. To top it all off, she's probably vomiting and has diarrhea.

Treatment of leptospirosis requires hospitalization for a couple of reasons. First, in addition to needing antibiotics to knock out the bacteria and other medications to control the vomiting and diarrhea, a dog with advanced symptoms will have lost a lot of fluid and need to have them replaced. Second, leptospirosis is a zoonotic disease, meaning it can be spread to people. Dogs with leptospirosis must be handled carefully to prevent infection. Even when your dog recovers, she can still be a carrier for up to a year. Your veterinarian can advise you on how to prevent infection after she's well.

Parvovirus. A highly contagious disease, parvovirus can be spread on an infected dog's paws, fur, saliva, and stool. It can also be carried on people's shoes and in crates or bedding used by infected dogs. Puppies younger than five months are hit especially hard by parvovirus and are most likely to die. Doberman Pinchers, Rottweilers, and Pitbulls are especially susceptible to parvovirus. The signs of parvovirus start to appear three to fourteen days after a dog has been exposed to it. Parvovirus can take two forms: The more common form is characterized by severe diarrhea, and the other rare form by damage to the heart muscle.

A dog with parvovirus is literally one sick puppy. If the disease affects her intestines, she'll be severely depressed with vomiting, abdominal pain, high fever, bloody diarrhea and—not surprisingly—no appetite. Few diseases cause this wide a range of serious symptoms. When parvo attacks the heart, young pups stop nursing and have trouble breathing. Usually they die quickly, but even if they recover they are likely to have congestive heart failure, which eventually kills them.

Vaccinations are available for parvovirus, but between six weeks and five months of age, pups are especially vulnerable to the disease, even if they've been vaccinated. The reason is complicated. You see, at birth, puppies get their immunities passively, through their mother's milk. Whatever diseases the mom has had or has been vaccinated against, the puppies get protection from, too. The effect of these maternal antibodies fades after weaning but may still be strong enough to interfere with the action of the parvovirus vaccine. With neither type of protection at full strength, the virus can slip in and do its dirty work. Even still, this does not mean you should put off getting a puppy vaccinated against parvo—two types of protection less-than-full strength is better than only one or none at all.

Parvovirus is hard to kill. The virus can last weeks to months in the environment. If your dog has had parvo, thoroughly disinfect everything she was in contact with, using one part chlorine bleach mixed with 30 parts water.

Rabies. That Harper Lee sure could tell a story. Her description of a dog with rabies in the Pulitzer Prize-winning book *To Kill a Mockingbird* is not only medically accurate, it conveys all the fear and danger of this dreaded disease. Of course, she was hardly the first to write about it: Rabies has been known for thousands of years and is mentioned in the legal tablets of Mesopotamia and in the writings of Aristotle and Xenophon. Some areas of the world—notably Australia, Great Britain, Iceland, Japan, and the Scandinavian nations—have managed to eliminate rabies through strict quarantines on incoming animals, but it is found everywhere else in the world.

The rabies virus is a bullet-shaped killer. It enters the body through an open wound, usually in the saliva delivered during a bite. It can infect—and kill—any warm-blooded animal, including human beings. Depending on the area of the country, the wild animals most likely to transmit rabies are raccoons, skunks, bats, and foxes. In 1995, out of a total of 7,881 reported cases of rabies, 146 cases were reported in dogs and 288 cases reported in cats.

Rabies takes two forms. One is described as furious and the other called paralytic. Paralytic rabies is usually the final stage, ending in death. A dog in the furious stage of rabies, which can last for one to seven days, goes through a range of behaviors. She can be restless or nervous, vicious, excitable, and sensitive to light and touch. Her breathing is heavy and fast, causing her to foam at the mouth. Another sign of rabies is a "personality change." For instance, a friendly dog might become withdrawn and snappish, or a shy dog might become much friendlier than usual. As the rabies virus does its work on the central nervous system, the animal has trouble walking and moving.

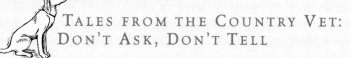

TALES FROM THE COUNTRY VET: DON'T ASK, DON'T TELL

Of all my early adventures and misadventures as a new DVM, there are a few that stand out. I'm sure I'll never forget my first case of suspected rabies.

The Wakeman family had been farming the same stretch of land for five generations. Among their prize possessions were their line of bulldogs, which great-grandpa Eustis Wakeman had begun in the previous century. One very hot July day, I was called out to the Wakeman farm on an emergency: One by one over the course of three days, an entire litter of Wakeman bulldogs and their mother had gone into convulsions and died. I examined the deceased dogs and could find nothing to explain their sudden demise. I knew all too well what had to happen next.

"Mr. Wakeman, we're going to have to check these dogs to make sure it wasn't rabies that killed them," I told the skeptical farmer. "It's not likely, but it's just too serious a public health threat. We have to have them tested . . . to rule it out."

"Alright, boy," he drawled. "Go ahead'n test." I swallowed hard. "Well, I'll have to take them to the lab . . . and the veterinary school . . . upstate." "Then take 'em," the farmer told me. "Well, the thing is . . . I don't need the whole dog. If it's rabies, it would be in the brain and spine, and so we just need . . ."

"Hold 'er right there, son," Mr. Wakeman said with a wave of his hand. "I appreciate you've had a lot of learnin' to get where you've got to, but there's no need to share all too much of it with me."

While it's bad form to approach any wild animal or strange dog, never try to approach one who is behaving oddly or having trouble with locomotion. You should even be extremely cautious around any animal you know who is acting erratically.

Because rabies is fatal, public health veterinarians recommend euthanizing any animal with signs of rabies who has bitten someone. A dog who appears healthy but has bitten someone must be kept confined for ten days to see if signs of rabies develop. An unvaccinated dog who's exposed to rabies must be strictly confined for six months, with a rabies vaccination given one month before she's released from quarantine—or euthanized. If a vaccinated dog is exposed to rabies, she should be given a booster shot immediately, confined, and closely observed for 90 days. Unfortunately, the only surefire way to confirm a dog has rabies is to examine her brain (specifically, the tissue of her central nervous system)—which means the dog can't be alive. If you have a dog or cat who dies rather suddenly—particularly after displaying unusual behavior—call your veterinarian immediately to see if you should have the animal checked for rabies.

Rabies is serious business. To protect your dog from rabies, you should have her vaccinated when she is three months old, again a year later, and once every three years afterward. If you are bitten by a rabid animal—or by any animal you can't confirm for certain doesn't have rabies—immediately clean the bite wound thoroughly with soap and water. Then call your doctor for immediate treatment, which may include a series of rabies vaccinations.

CAN I CATCH IT FROM MY DOG?: ZOONOTIC CONDITIONS

We can't catch colds from our dogs, but they can share other diseases with us. Conditions that can be spread from dogs to humans are called zoonotic diseases. Some are merely unpleasant, such as the ringworm fungus, but others like salmonella poisoning or rabies can have more serious consequences. Dogs can also pass along leptospirosis, known as Weil's disease in humans, as well as parasites such as scabies, round-worms, tapeworms, hookworms, and the tick-borne Lyme disease and Rocky Mountain spotted fever.

Fortunately, it's not too difficult to prevent Ginger from spreading any diseases to us. She can be vaccinated against leptospirosis and rabies, of course. Worms can be kept under control by picking up her stool regularly and having regular fecal exams and deworming as needed. Good hygiene—yours, that is—is one of the most important ways you can prevent zoonosis. So be sure to wash your hands thoroughly after handling the dog or picking up after her. This is especially important to remember for young children, elderly or debilitated people, and people with immune system disorders or undergoing cancer chemotherapy, all of whom are most susceptible to zoonotic diseases.

Ticks. If you live in a wooded or grassy area or take your dog to such places, examine Rover daily for ticks during warm weather. You're most likely to find ticks between her toes or on her head, neck, or ears. Remove ticks with tweezers, grasping them near the tick's head and pulling slowly but firmly. Be careful not to touch the ticks your-self. In fact, it's probably a good idea to wear rubber gloves when you're removing them. Drop ticks in a jar of rubbing alcohol to kill them. Other folk methods—coating the tick with gasoline or petro-leum jelly, or burning it—are more likely to complicate matters and can actually be very dangerous if the tick bursts or the dog's hair catches fire. However, it can help to spray the dog with a flea-and-tick insecticide before removing the little blood-suckers. Newer tick-control prescription products are very effective at controlling ticks; check with your vet for a prescription.

Lyme disease and Rocky Mountain spotted fever. Lyme disease is spread by the bite of ticks carrying the slender spiraling bacteria called *Borrelia burgdorferi spirochete*. Ticks carrying Lyme disease include the deer tick in the eastern United States and the western black-legged tick on the West Coast. Ticks come out primarily in the spring and summer, especially when it's rainy, so Lyme disease is most common during the months of May through August, usually reaching a high in July. Most cases are found in the Northeast and mid-Atlantic, but Lyme disease has been reported in most of the lower 48 states.

When dogs get Lyme disease, it usually shows up in the form of arthritis. Suddenly they're lame because their joints are tender and swollen. Not surprisingly, they're listless and weak, don't feel like eating, and may have a fever. In severe cases, Lyme disease can affect the heart, kidneys, and nervous system.

Unfortunately, Lyme disease is difficult to diagnose and is often confused with other diseases. If the dog has been bitten by ticks, develops the signs described above, and then responds to antibiotics, it's a pretty safe bet she was suffering from Lyme disease. If you live in an area where ticks are pretty common, ask your vet for advice on keeping them at bay with flea-and-tick-killing sprays, powders, and collars, or with the Lyme disease vaccine.

Rocky Mountain spotted fever, also spread by contact with ticks, is caused by a different kind of bacteria called a rickettsia, which is rod-shaped and multiplies only within the cells of its host. Wood ticks and American dog ticks are the carriers of Rocky Mountain spotted fever, which is most common in the plains of the Midwest and in the mid-Atlantic states.

A dog with Rocky Mountain spotted fever has—of course—a fever, painful joints, and no appetite. In people, Rocky Mountain spotted fever causes flulike symptoms: fever, chills, achy muscles, nausea, and vomiting. They may be sensitive to light, and a rash develops on their hands, wrists, ankles, and feet, sometimes spreading to the rest of the body. As with Lyme disease, antibiotics are the treatment of choice. Again, the best offense is a good defense: Examine your dog regularly for ticks, remove them carefully when you find them, and use insecticidal products that will kill or repel them.

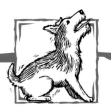

At-Home Health Care: Emergencies and First Aid

Have you ever seen a dog injured in a fight or hit by a car? Perhaps you could only shake your head and walk away. Not because you didn't care, but because you didn't know how to help the dog. What if your dog was involved in an emergency situation? Would you know what to do? Since your dog depends on you, you need to be prepared.

This chapter helps you handle simple first aid to keep your pet alive until you can get him to the vet. From bleeding to shock, you'll learn what you can do at home to help your pet. Practice these techniques ahead of time so that you'll know how to handle the emergency when it actually happens. Remember, every minute counts.

First Aid

In most cases, the first person to take care of your dog in an emergency will be you. When you have your dog's life in your hands, you need to act quickly and confidently. Here are some emergency situations and techniques to stabilize your dog and keep things under control until the vet can take over.

Bleeding

Bright-red blood spurting from a wound means an artery (one of the main blood pathways) is involved. A slower stream of dark-red blood suggests the injury involves a smaller vein. To help stop bleeding of any kind, apply direct pressure with a gauze pad, handkerchief, or other clean cloth. Secure the pad or have someone hold it in place, and get veterinary help right away. Bleeding from cuts on the ear, paw pad, or penis is particularly hard to control, so apply direct pressure and call the vet immediately.

Sometimes dogs get little scratches or scrapes that bleed. These don't require a trip to the vet, but they should still be treated. Clean up the injury with three-percent hydrogen peroxide solution. When the wound stops bleeding, you can apply antibiotic ointment.

You can also cover a wound with a bandage. Use gauze bandages or whatever clean cloth is available to wrap the wound. Wrap an adhesive bandage over the top of the cloth or bandage, and secure it with medical adhesive tape. Wrap the tape loosely so that it doesn't stick to your dog's fur. For a foot bandage that's quick and easy to change, place a gauze pad over the wound, cover it with a baby sock, and secure it with tape.

Broken Bones

Sometimes broken bones (or fractures) are easy to spot: a bend in a leg where it doesn't usually bend, a foot pointing at an unnatural angle. Compound fractures are even more obvious, since part of the

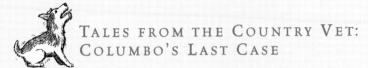

TALES FROM THE COUNTRY VET: COLUMBO'S LAST CASE

Marylou named her Bloodhound Columbo, after the tenacious television detective. True to his namesake, Columbo did his fair share of snooping around the yard. One afternoon, a frantic Marylou called me at the office.

"Columbo has been pacing and whining," she told me, the worry evident in her voice. "He keeps trying to throw up, but all that comes up is a lot of saliva. I could swear his stomach is bigger, so I measured it an hour ago. I measured it again just a minute ago, and it was an inch bigger. That's when I called."

I took a deep breath. "I think you already suspect what might be going on, Marylou," I told her. "You've been around these dogs long enough to know the signs of bloat when you see them." I heard Marylou gasp. "That's what I was afraid of," she said, choking back tears. "There's not much hope for him, is there?"

Bloat is a term that describes the sudden distended abdomen that can occur in large-breed dogs, typically those with deep chests such as Bloodhounds, Doberman Pinschers, or Saint

bone protrudes through the skin. But even if your dog is just limping badly or has taken a hard knock and has an area that seems very sore to the touch, you could be dealing with a cracked or broken bone. In any of these cases, try to keep the dog as still as possible; activity can turn a simple break into a compound fracture. Wrap the dog in a blanket to help keep him from going into shock; and get veterinary help immediately.

Bernards. It's not completely clear exactly what causes bloat, but it kills as many as 50 percent to 60 percent of the dogs who get it. The telltale abdominal bloating is the result of gastric torsion—the stomach gets twisted, trapping gas and fluid, and shutting off digestion. A common scenario for gastric torsion in at-risk dogs is a large meal, followed by a period of activity.

I wanted to reassure Marylou but still be realistic. I told her to meet me at the clinic—and to keep up her courage. Ten minutes later, I had Columbo on the examining table. Twenty minutes later, I had successfully inserted a stomach tube and released the trapped gas and fluids. "It looks like everything's going to be fine," I said happily to a much relieved Marylou. "If I hadn't been able to get the tube in, we'd have had to open him up—a much more risky procedure, and not guaranteed to be successful.

"I know you like to send Columbo out snooping around in the yard after dinner, but my advice to you is to feed him a couple of smaller meals during the day, don't let him drink a large amount of water at one time... and retire him from the after-meals police work."

Be extra careful if your dog seems to be paralyzed or if his legs are stiff or limp—these are the signs of a spinal cord injury. Move him only as much as you have to. You can make a stretcher with a board or a rigid piece of cardboard large enough to support his back. If nothing else is available, use a blanket pulled taut. Try to slide the dog onto the stretcher instead of lifting him. Place one hand under the dog's chest and the other under his rear; carefully lift or slide the dog onto the

board. Tie the dog to
the board, and keep
his back, head, and
forelegs still
during the ride to
the veterinary hospital.

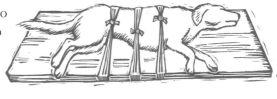

Head injuries—most notably when a dog is hit by a car—may result
in a broken jaw or fractured skull. Although a skull fracture isn't obvious, a broken jaw is usually indicated by the lower jaw hanging open
and drooling. Place a scarf or bandage beneath the dog's chin and tie it
behind his ears to immobilize the jaw. A dog with a fractured skull
may be dizzy or unconscious, and sometimes has a bloody nose. In
both cases, carefully control any bleeding, and get the dog to a vet
right away.

Burns

A curious dog, especially a puppy, will stick his nose into all kinds of
trouble, including hot stoves or fireplaces. If your dog's paws or fur
get singed, use cool water or a cool compress to soothe the area. A
burn over a large area of the body should be covered with a thick layer
of cloth or gauze (cotton balls or cotton batting will stick to the skin,
so don't use them). Wrap the dog in a blanket to keep him warm so
he won't go into shock, and get veterinary help right away. After a
minor burn has had a couple of days to heal, you can apply the juice
of an aloe leaf to help soothe the pain.

Some old wives' tales suggest using butter, ointment, or ice to soothe
and heal a burn, but these can only make matters worse. Butter and
ointment may take away some of the discomfort, but they slow down
healing. Ice also numbs pain but can do further damage to the skin.

By the way, fire isn't the only cause of burns. Dogs also get chemical
burns from items such as battery acid and common household prod-

ucts such as bleach and toilet bowl cleaners. When giving your dog first aid for a chemical burn, follow the same general advice as for fire burns, but be sure to protect your hands and eyes so you don't get injured, too. Again, take your dog to the vet for further treatment as soon as possible.

Electrical burns typically occur when a bored or curious dog decides to gnaw on an electrical cord. These burns are tricky to treat since they will mostly be around the corners of the mouth or on the tongue and palate. If the electrical shock is severe, he might have a seizure or lose consciousness; his breathing could slow down; and his heart could even stop beating. In some cases edema (fluid) builds up in the lungs, causing difficulty in breathing, which is very serious. If you find your dog in this condition, be sure to switch off the electrical source before you touch him. Then get him to the vet immediately.

CHOKING

Lacking thumbs and fingers, dogs pick up interesting items with their mouths. Of course, anything that goes into your dog's mouth may end up being chewed and swallowed. Items such as chicken bones, razor blades, and small toys may not make it all the way down the throat, resulting in choking. If your dog exhibits signs of choking—including coughing, gagging, and pawing at his mouth—force his mouth open by pressing the thumb and forefingers of one hand into the dog's upper cheeks and pulling downward on the lower jaw. Gently try to remove any caught object with your fingers or a pair of needle-nose pliers. If that doesn't work, you can try using the Heimlich maneuver. Standing over or behind the dog, wrap your arms around his abdomen and give a quick squeeze. Continue this procedure until the object pops out. (Note: The Heimlich maneuver isn't effective on objects that become embedded in the dog's throat, such as splintered chicken bones.) Once the object is removed, or if you aren't able to get it out, get your dog to the vet right away.

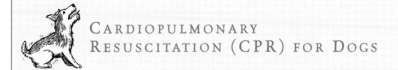

CARDIOPULMONARY RESUSCITATION (CPR) FOR DOGS

If your dog stops breathing and his heart stops beating, you have just a matter of minutes to save his life. Unless you live upstairs from the veterinarian, those first crucial minutes will be in your hands. That's why every dog owner should know canine CPR.

First, check the dog's breathing and pulse or heartbeat. To feel for his heartbeat, hold your fingers firmly against his chest on the left side just below his elbow. You can feel for you dog's pulse by placing your fingers on his inner thigh. If you can feel a pulse or heartbeat, do not give CPR—get the dog to a vet immediately, checking on your dog along the way. If there's no heartbeat or pulse, lay the dog on his side on the floor or some other flat, hard surface. Begin CPR by using the palm of your hand to compress the

DROWNING

Even though we've all heard of the doggie paddle and have seen retrievers splashing happily after toys and downed birds, dogs aren't born as expert swimmers. Many dogs drown every year from tumbles out of boats, off of piers, and into backyard swimming pools. Unless your dog is an experienced swimmer, an unexpected dip into water over his head (and for most dogs, that's only a foot or two deep) can have tragic results. Even a dog who's used to playing at the beach can lower part of the chest, directly behind the front legs (this is where the heart is located) with six quick, firm squeezes. The amount of pressure you use depends on the size of the dog. Stop for five seconds, then continue. Between the series of chest compressions, have a helper provide artificial respiration.

To start artificial respiration, look in the dog's mouth and clear away anything that might be blocking the airway. Make sure the tongue is pulled forward; then wrap your hands around the dog's muzzle so the seal around his lips is airtight. Stretch his head and neck forward, and blow steadily into his nostrils for three seconds. If you are successful, the chest will expand. Release the muzzle so the air can come out, then continue until the dog is breathing on his own.

quickly get into trouble if he falls into a swimming pool and can't get up over the slippery side. Deep or cold lake water or a moment's confusion or panic can also get a dog out past his limit of exhaustion. When a swimming dog tires, he drowns.

With this in mind, never leave your dog unattended near any pool or body of water. And even when you're there, you should be ready and able to go into the water after your dog if he needs you. Once you get him out of the water, check to see if he's breathing. Look at the dog's gums; if they're blue or gray, he's not getting enough oxygen, even if he appears to be breathing. If your dog isn't breathing, lift him up with his head facing down and thump the sides of his chest. This will help drain water out of the airways. You may have to give artificial respiration to get him breathing. (See the section on CPR for dogs in this chapter.) Once he's breathing, get your dog to the vet. Water inhaled into the lungs can cause a serious form of pneumonia.

FROSTBITE

Frostbite occurs when the skin becomes partially or totally frozen. The parts of a dog most likely to become frostbitten are the ear tips, toes or paw pads, and tail. If he has a good, sturdy shelter, your dog probably won't get frostbite, but he is more prone to it if he's very young, very old, or not in the best of health. The skin of a dog with frostbite is pale, later reddening and becoming hot and painful when touched. Sometimes the skin swells and peels. If your dog has frostbite, keep him warm to ward off shock but thaw the skin out slowly with warm, moist towels, changing them often. You can make things worse by rubbing the skin briskly or using hot towels. When the skin color looks normal again, you can stop warming it. Get veterinary help as soon as possible.

HEAT EXHAUSTION AND HEATSTROKE

A dog has only a few sweat glands, so his body's cooling system is not as efficient as ours. So if heatstroke or heat exhaustion is a risk for people during heavy exertion or on hot or humid days, it's that much more likely for a dog. Typical scenarios of heat-related problems in dogs are overdoing it with play in warm weather, going jogging with a human friend, and being left in a closed car on hot or sunny days.

A dog with heat exhaustion might collapse, vomit, or have muscle cramps and often has an elevated body temperature. Get him someplace cool or shady, and cool him off by sponging his head and shoulders with cool—not cold—water. In a case of heatstroke, the dog's body-temperature control mechanism is out of whack. He starts panting hard, and his breathing is loud and raspy. His temperature can shoot up to 106 degrees Fahrenheit or more, and his gums sometimes turn purple or gray, a sign he's not getting enough oxygen. In severe cases, the dog's throat can swell, cutting off his air. Dogs with short noses, like Pugs, Bulldogs, or Boston Terriers, are especially prone to heatstroke. Cool the dog down the way you would for heat exhaustion, but if his gums have changed color, get him to a vet right away. If possible, bring someone along to sponge him down in the car.

Preventing heat exhaustion or heatstroke is simply a matter of good old-fashioned common sense. Limit a dog's activity during the hottest part of the day, watch him for signs of tiring during play or runs, and make sure he always has access to shade and lots of cool, fresh water.

POISONING

In the dog's view of the universe, everything fits into one of three categories: food, another dog, or something else. In their quest to figure out if an item fits into the first category, dogs pick up—and swallow—all sorts of things. Household cleansers, rat poisons, and yard treatments are just a few of the things dogs get into—with toxic consequences. A number of common household plants should also be marked with the skull-and-crossbones poison symbol, including seasonal plants such as Easter lilies, as well as azaleas, caladium, dumbcane (dieffenbachia), English ivy (berries and leaves), ficus (leaves), holly, mistletoe (berries), oleander, and philodendron. Many bulbs—amaryllis, daffodil, iris, and tulip—are also poisonous. Signs of poisoning include drooling or vomiting, seizure, diarrhea, or collapse for no other apparent reason. A dog who has been poisoned may also have muscular weakness, and his eyes, mouth, or skin might seem irritated.

If you think your dog has eaten something poisonous, your first instinct may be to get it out of him as quickly as possible. Many of us

CALLING A POISON HOTLINE

If you can't get to a veterinarian, check your first aid book or call the National Animal Poison Control Center (NAPCC). Be ready with your name, address, and phone number; information about the poison (how much was consumed, how long since it happened); your dog's breed, age, sex, and weight; and what signs your dog is showing (vomiting, seizures, muscle tremors, diarrhea, difficulty breathing, skin irritation, drooling, weakness, abdominal pain, paralysis).

The Animal Poison Hotline of the NAPCC is operated by the University of Illinois College of Veterinary Medicine (2001 South Lincoln Avenue, Urbana, Illinois 61801). There is a charge for calls, and you have two options for payment and fees:

• Call 1 (888) 4ANIHELP or 1 (800) 548-2423. There's a $30 flat fee, chargeable to a credit card (have your charge card ready).

• Call 1 (900) 680-0000. The charge is $20 for the first five minutes, $2.95 per minute thereafter; charges will appear on your next phone bill.

were taught to induce vomiting in cases of poisoning—but in most instances, doing so can just make the situation worse. So before you induce vomiting, call the vet or animal poison control center for advice. (Note: Some toxic products have advice on whether or not to induce vomiting printed right on the package.)

As a general rule, vomiting should not be induced for moderate to strong acids (toilet bowl cleaner, chlorine, battery acid) or alkali (drain cleaners, dishwashing detergent). Instead, for acids, give an antacid such as Milk of Magnesia, at a dosage of one teaspoon for each five pounds of the dog's body weight. For an alkali, give one to five teaspoons (depending on your dog's size) of vinegar or lemon juice. Check your pet first aid kit for activated charcoal tablets and give the recommended dosage to your dog. Any poison still in the dog's stomach will bind to the charcoal instead of spreading through the body.

Next, get your dog to the vet right away. Bring the package containing the poison if you know what it is. If your dog has thrown up, bring a sample of the vomit (it can help your vet figure out what the dog has eaten). If a veterinarian is not available but you can identify the substance, call the National Animal Poison Control Center.

If your vet does recommend you induce vomiting, you can use ¼ to one teaspoon of syrup of ipecac; one part three-percent hydrogen peroxide mixed with one part water (give one to two teaspoons of the mixture); or mix one teaspoon to one tablespoon of dry mustard with one cup of water. To administer the mixture, tip your dog's head slightly backward. Pull the lower lip out at the corner to make a pouch. Using a plastic eyedropper, place the fluid slowly into the pouch a little at a time. Allow each small amount to be swallowed before giving any more of the dose. Gently rub the throat to stimulate the swallowing. Don't induce vomiting if your dog is unconscious or seems very depressed, if he's swallowed something sharp, such as razor blades or glass, or if it has been more than two hours since he was poisoned.

Not all poisoning happens by mouth. Some poisons are absorbed through the skin, especially the feet. If your dog walks in something toxic or gets it on his coat and skin, protect your hands with rubber gloves and rinse him thoroughly with warm water—then get veterinary help as soon as possible.

In any case of poisoning, prompt action and fast, expert advice may be the difference between life and death. Be absolutely certain a conscious dog suspected of being poisoned gets plenty of water to drink. The water will dilute the poison in his digestive system.

SHOCK

Shock is the body's response to a major trauma or injury such as being hit by a car, heavy blood or fluid loss, or poisoning. Knowing it's in trouble, the body shifts into low gear, which actually helps the victim survive the immediate danger. If it's not treated, however, shock can be fatal because the body isn't able to maintain the necessary blood pressure. A dog who's in shock might have a weak, rapid pulse; dry gums; pale or gray lips; shallow, rapid breathing; or a lower-than-normal temperature. If he's bleeding, get it under control. Keep the dog still and warm, and get him to a vet right away.

SNAKEBITE

Wherever you live in the continental United States, poisonous snakes can pose problems for curious dogs. Dogs are most likely to get bitten on the nose or head, followed by the front legs. The Eastern diamondback rattlesnake is the most venomous of snakes in this country, but many dogs have also died from the bite of a cottonmouth snake.

If you're not sure whether the snake that bit your dog is poisonous, look at the marks left by the bite. A harmless snake leaves horseshoe-shaped teeth marks, while a venomous one leaves the telltale fang marks. Even if you didn't see the snake or can't clearly determine the pattern of the bite, severe swelling at the bite site, extreme pain, and, slow, steady bleeding are all signs of a venomous bite.

A massive dose of venom can bring your dog to the point of death quickly, and you may have to give CPR before you can get him to the vet. Don't use ice or a tourniquet on the wound, and don't try to suck the venom out. Carry him to the car or to help if possible; allowing him to walk will just spread the poison more quickly.

Taking a Dog's Temperature

Elevated body temperature is a sign of disease, heat exhaustion, and heatstroke. To take your dog's temperature, use a rectal thermometer (glass or electronic) lubricated with petroleum jelly, K-Y jelly, or vegetable oil. With the dog lying flat, lift the tail and gently insert the thermometer into his rectum. It's a good idea to have someone else restrain the dog so she can't escape. Leave the thermometer in for one or two minutes, then remove it to read the temperature. A dog's normal temperature ranges from 100 to 102.5 degrees Fahrenheit, with smaller dogs tending to have higher temperatures. Call your veterinarian if the temperature is below 100 degrees Fahrenheit or higher than 103 degrees Fahrenheit.

Moving and Handling an Injured Dog

Even the most mild-mannered dog can—and will—bite if he's hurt and scared. Many owners make the mistake of believing they can just scoop up their injured dog and carry him to safety. That's true—but only if the owner is willing to run the risk of some serious bites. Insead, always take steps to protect yourself before you start any first-aid procedures on your dog. After all, if you end up getting hurt, you might not be able to help him.

Before doing anything with an injured dog, it's a good idea to muzzle him. This prevents misunderstandings and sudden snapping if you touch a painful area. You can keep a dog muzzle in your first-aid kit or improvise one as needed using pantyhose, a necktie, or some other strip of cloth. Simply wrap the fabric around the dog's muzzle, loop it, and tie the ends behind the dog's head to hold it in place. (Do not put a muzzle on a dog who is vomiting or can not breathe through his nose.)

Go slowly when moving a dog with a broken bone or possible spinal injury. Keep the broken limb as still as possible and try to surround the dog with padding for the car ride to the veterinary hospital. For a dog with a possible spinal injury, even more care is needed to prevent severing the spinal cord—move him as little as possible. Put together a makeshift stretcher with a board, a sturdy piece of cardboard, or even a baking sheet for a small dog. (To make a stretcher, see the section on broken bones in this chapter.) If nothing else is available, you can put the dog on a blanket, pull it tight at the ends, and carry him that way.

Here are some other tried-and-true restraining techniques:

- If your dog is small, you can restrain him with a towel. Simply wrap a large towel around the dog's neck and hold the towel in front of his head. If necessary, gently pin the towel in place.

- For smaller dogs, grasp the dog by his collar and place your other arm over his back and around his body. At the same time, pull forward on the collar and lift the dog's body, cradling it against your body.

- For larger dogs, slip one arm under his neck, holding his throat in the crook of your arm. Make sure the dog can breathe easily. Place your other arm under his stomach. Lift with both arms.

- If the dog is very large, slip one arm under his neck, holding his chest in the crook of your arm. Again, make sure the dog can breathe easily. Place your other arm under the dog's rump and, pressing your arms toward one another, lift the dog.

To help prevent shock, wrap the dog in a blanket to keep him warm. And stay calm. Moving and speaking calmly and confidently will reassure your dog and help him relax.

YOUR HOME VETERINARY FIRST-AID KIT

Ready-made first-aid kits are available at pet stores or through catalogs. You can also put one together yourself, using items from around the house. Put the kit where it can be easily found and include your veterinarian's business card, along with the phone number for and directions to the nearest emergency clinic. Check the kit every once in a while to make sure you aren't running low on any supplies and everything is still usable. The following items make up a basic first-aid kit:

- Activated charcoal (available at drugstores) for absorbing poisons

- Adhesive tape to secure bandages

- Antibacterial ointment or powder for cleaning wounds

- Antidiarrheal agent such as Kaopectate (Ask your vet what amount is appropriate for controlling your dog's diarrhea.)

- Blunt-tipped scissors to trim away hair from wounds and cut bandaging material

- Cotton balls and cotton swabs

- Gauze pads and rolls to make bandages

- Three-percent hydrogen peroxide to clean wounds

- K-Y jelly or petroleum jelly to lubricate a thermometer

- Laxative or antacid such as Milk of Magnesia

- Needleless syringe for giving liquid medications

- Plaster splint for broken limbs

- Plastic eyedropper to administer liquid medications or eyedrops

- Rectal thermometer

- Rubbing alcohol

- Syrup of ipecac to induce vomiting

- Tweezers

Other helpful items for your kit might be needle-nose pliers to remove porcupine quills or other items stuck in the mouth or throat, sanitary napkins to help stop heavy blood flow, and towels.

YOUR DOG'S RECOVERY AT HOME

Any time your dog needs treatment for a significant health problem, his recovery at home will go faster if he gets lots of tender loving nursing care. It's up to you to make sure he gets plenty of rest, eats right, takes all his medicine, and doesn't get too active too soon.

Make him a comfortable bed in a quiet area away from all the hubbub in your home. This could be in a bedroom, a laundry room, or a bathroom that isn't used often. If you have kids in your household, don't let the them bother the dog too much. They can go in one at a time for a few minutes each day to sit quietly with Rex, but no rough-housing or loud sounds until he's feeling better.

To tempt his tastebuds, serve his food warm—but not so hot he burns his mouth—or top it with something that smells good, such as chicken or beef broth. Scrambled eggs, yogurt, and cottage cheese will also encourage his appetite. Be sure to check with your vet before supplementing his diet to make sure you aren't offering anything he shouldn't have. Rex will need plenty of fresh, cool water as well. Make it easy for him to reach so he'll get enough.

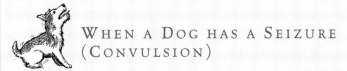

WHEN A DOG HAS A SEIZURE (CONVULSION)

Seizures, or convulsions, look scary, but when a dog has a seizure, it's usually harder on the owner watching helplessly than on the dog. Seizures may occur in response to poisons, infection, nervous system disorders, or injuries, especially to the head. Epilepsy is a neurological problem that can cause repeated seizures but can be controlled with medication.

Most seizures aren't painful, and despite the old wives' tale, the dog is not going to swallow his tongue. So don't try to put your fingers in the mouth of a dog having a seizure, unless you want to leave them behind. Instead, protect the dog from accidental injury by wrapping him in a blanket until the seizure is over. Most seizures last only a minute or two at most (although it seems much longer for the owner). To help you get through your dog's seizure, watch him carefully—even take notes. Report everything to the vet, which will help in diagnosis. Your vet will want to know whether the dog thrashed about or became stiff; whether he lost consciousness or didn't seem to recognize you; if he acted strangely just before the seizure; if his muscles twitched at the beginning of the seizure; and how long the seizure lasted.

Follow your veterinarian's directions to the letter when it comes to exercise. If your dog is recovering from surgery, especially for a broken bone, it's important he doesn't overdo it. It's hard to keep a good dog down, but if you want him to recover properly, you'll have to be lovingly firm.

Finally, even if he seems to be well, don't stop giving Rex all his prescribed medications until they're all gone. Looks can be deceiving, and it's most likely he needs all the healing power the full course of medication contains. Before you take your pooch home from the vet or animal hospital, ask the doctor or a technician to show you how to give the medication properly. Dogs can be pretty sneaky about hiding pills under their tongues or in their cheeks and spitting them out later. The pros can show you some tried-and-true tricks to outsmart even the cagiest canine.

GIVING DOGS MEDICATIONS

If you've been a dog owner for awhile, you know that getting Fido to take his medicine is not always easy. Rare is the dog who will take his medicine willingly, so here are some helpful ways to give your dog his medicine at home.

Pills. If you're fortunate, you may have one of those dogs who will actually take pills without any fuss at all. For others, it may be easiest to have someone else hold the dog while you give him the pill. With practice, though, most owners can perfect the technique enough to pill their dogs solo.

Be sure you have the pill out and ready to go before you start. Hold the dog's head firmly with one hand or, if he's small, hold him firmly between your knees while kneeling on the floor. If you're working with a puppy or a toy breed, it might be easier to wrap the dog in a towel so he can't move, or place him on a table or counter. Hold the pill in your right hand (reverse these directions if you are left-handed). Using the first and middle fingers of your left hand, gently open Fido's jaws, and put the pill as far back on the tongue as you can get it. Close his mouth and stroke his throat to get the pill to go down.

Another way to give pills is to tilt Fido's head straight up with your left hand. Hold the pill between the thumb and forefinger of your right hand, and use the middle finger to open his mouth. Put the pill into the back of his mouth, and use your forefinger to push it over the tongue. To get him to swallow, hold his mouth closed and rub or blow into his nose.

> Store all medications for your dog in a cool place since heat can spoil their effectiveness.

If all else fails, disguise the pill by wrapping it in something soft and tasty such as cream cheese or peanut butter. Unless Fido is really smart or really cautious about what he puts into his mouth, the pill will go down without him even knowing it. Since some medications need to be given on an empty stomach, interact with certain foods, or should not be accidentally chewed, be sure to ask your veterinarian if it's okay to give the pill this way.

Liquid medications. Again, get the medicine ready: Shake the bottle if needed, measure the dosage, and fill the dropper. Now get the dog. Hold him the same way you would if you were giving a pill. With his head tilted upward, pry open his mouth and aim the eyedropper at the cheek pouch. Then, with the dropper still inside, hold his mouth closed, and squeeze out the medication. He'll swallow automatically when the liquid reaches the back of his mouth. Make sure he has swallowed before you release your hold on his mouth. Just to be on the safe side, rub or blow into his nose to make him lick, which will trigger swallowing.

Ear drops. Get a good grasp on the dog. Holding his ear gently but firmly, tilt his head slightly to the opposite side. Drop the correct dosage into the ear and gently fold the ear down or together and rub the cartilage at the base of his ear to get the medication all the way into the ear canal. This also helps keep more of the medicine in the dog's ear if your dog shakes his head afterward.

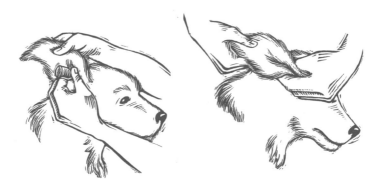

Eyedrops. Get everything ready and measure out the proper dosage. Restrain the dog gently but firmly. It's especially important to keep his head still so the medicine goes in his eye but the dropper doesn't. Hold the dropper in your right hand (reverse this if you are left-handed), tilt his head up and aim the drops at the inner corner of the eye, directly on the eyeball. Don't touch the eye with the tip of the eye-dropper. To make sure the medication gets distributed evenly over the eye, close and open the eyelid.

Ointments. Sometimes ointments are prescribed for the eyes or ears. To apply ointment to the eyes, hold Fido's head steady, and gently pull down on his lower lid, exposing the inner eyelid. Put the ointment on the inside lower lid. Be careful not to get it directly on the eyeball. You can also pull the upper lid back and put the ointment on the white of the eye. To make sure the medication gets distributed evenly over the eye, close and open the eyelid. To apply ointments to ears, follow the same directions for ear drops.

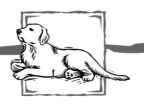

COMMON PHYSICAL PROBLEMS AND HOME REMEDIES

When you think of health care, you probably think of doctor visits and what's called "acute care"—medical treatment for illness or injury. But your dog can also have less serious problems that can be taken care of at home, either on your own or with a little help from your veterinarian. From fighting fleas to mending scrapes, you can do a lot to keep your dog healthy.

Here are a few tips for some of the most likely situations you'll run across, including what you can—and can't—do at home and when to call the vet. We'll also take a look at some alternative health care options, such as acupuncture and homeopathy, and how to handle your dog's golden years.

FLEAS

There's no doubt. Fleas can be the bane of a dog's (and dog owner's) existence. The little critters are pretty amazing. They've got six tiny legs and no wings, yet they can leap tall dogs in a single bound. Scientists have identified nearly 2,000 species of fleas, but ironically, it's *Ctenocephalides felis*—the cat flea—that gives dogs the most grief.

When one of his dogs comes up with fleas, my old pal, Hoke Mitchell, always leaves the same message at my office: "Attack of the tiny vampires. Send help immediately." It may be a joke (or Hoke's idea of a joke), but it makes two important points: Fleas are blood suckers, and where there's one, you can be certain there are a whole lot more. Besides the usual minor itching and scratching a flea infestation causes, some dogs are extra-sensitive to flea saliva. Just one bite may be enough to bring on the unbearable itching of flea-allergy dermatitis (FAD). In severe cases, the cycle of itching and scratching causes the dog's skin to thicken and her hair to fall out. The raw skin is also more vulnerable to bacterial infections.

Fortunately, there's a variety of well-tested and readily available products to kill or repel fleas. Borates (used in those powdered flea-control products you sprinkle on your carpets) cause adult fleas, eggs, and larvae to lose moisture and dry up. Insect growth regulators stop immature fleas from becoming adults and reproducing. New weapons in the war on fleas include lufenuron, the active ingredient in the recently developed flea-control pill that interferes with the flea egg's ability to hatch. Also, two products, introduced in 1996 under the brand names of Frontline and Advantage, work by disrupting the function of a flea's nervous system. Available only through veterinarians, they both kill adult fleas on contact and have long-lasting effects.

Whatever flea-control products you choose, always read and follow directions precisely. Never assume if a little is good, a lot will be better.

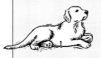

Natural Ways to Fight Fleas

If you're leery of using chemical products on your dog or home, there are a number of plant-, vitamin-, and herbal-based natural flea treatments available. Adding garlic or brewer's yeast to a dog's food has long been thought to help keep fleas from alighting and biting. Since both are ordinary food products and not harmful to dogs, there's really nothing to lose by giving them a try. Herbal flea collars and powders are also popular and widely available. Eucalyptus, fennel, rosemary, rue, wormwood, and yellow dock all seem to act as flea repellents. To make your own herbal flea powder, combine equal amounts of these herbs and mix them well. Sprinkle a small amount of the powder on your dog's coat and massage it in thoroughly, making sure to work it all the way down to the skin. You can also use a drop or two of the essential oils of eucalyptus and rosemary on a plain canvas or fabric-covered collar. As with any flea collar, though, watch for signs of hair loss or skin irritation around the neck, and be careful that the dog doesn't chew on the collar. You can also buy ready-made herbal flea collars at pet supply and natural food stores.

Every flea product (natural or other) is a poison of some kind, and, if used incorrectly, can be dangerous.

What to Do About It

Even with all the new safer and longer-lasting flea-control products available, you still need to follow some basic rules to the letter in order to get the upper hand with fleas.

Build a flea trap. While building a flea trap won't rid your house of fleas, it's a good way to verify that you've got them in your house and determine how severe an infestation you're dealing with. Hang a light source over a sticky, disposable surface (flypaper works well for this) or a bowl of soapy water. The heat from the light source attracts any nearby fleas, many of which will then get caught on the sticky surface or in the water. You'll notice the fleas as small, dark, flat-bodied insects, roughly the size of the commas in this sentence.

Give fleas an eviction notice. You absolutely must treat all dogs and cats, as well as the premises—all at the same time—and be diligent about follow-up treatment and future preventative treatment. Treat carpets with a borate-based powder. Spray the yard, too. Ideally, you should use an outdoor flea-control product that is long-lasting, kills adult fleas, and contains insect growth regulators to catch immature fleas before they can grow up and repopulate your property. Moist, shady areas are favorite flea playgrounds and breeding grounds, so clear out falled leaves, pine needles, wood, and garbage from under trees, shrubs, and plants. If spraying the whole grounds isn't feasible, try to at least concentrate on areas your dog frequents: around the doghouse, along the fence line, under the porch, and so on.

Professional pest-control companies can handle flea control for you. But before you sign the contract, get written information on the compounds and method of application the company uses. Run the list by your veterinarian.

Take your dog for a dip. Actually, the best thing to do with a dog who has fleas while the premises are being "de-fleaed" is to take her to the veterinarian for a medicated dip or other flea treatment. In fact, that's also a good idea for an effective flea-control program. Your vet may choose to give your dog lufenuron for flea control, which is given as a monthly pill. In warm areas like southern California, dogs on lufenuron get their pills year-round. In temperate areas of the country, where winter gets cold enough to kill off fleas, the pills are only given during flea season—from early spring to sometime in the fall. Talk to your vet about the options, though. It may be that one of the topical treatments works best for you and your dog. Topicals hit fleas right where they live—on the outside of your dog—and start working immediately. If your dog loves to swim or play in the water, or gets bathed frequently, a topical can get washed off, though. Newer topical products like Frontline have very long residual effects, only needing to be applied every two or three months, and they don't wash off. Fleas can develop resistance to a particular product in a surprisingly short time, so your veterinarian may recommend a program of alternating products and treatment strategies.

Treat hot spots. Dogs with flea-allergy dermatitis often develop hot spots—moist, infected areas of the skin. To soothe hot spots, mix one part melaleuca oil and one part water. Put the solution in a spray bottle, and use it whenever your dog is biting or scratching. You can also apply a natural menthol liniment such as Absorbine Jr. a few times a day until the area dries up.

WHEN TO CALL THE VET

Heavy drooling and a case of the shakes are the most likely early signs of chemical poisoning. If you see these symptoms in your dog—whether during the course of a flea-control program or not—get her to the vet immediately. Left untreated, chemical poisoning may quickly progress to convulsions, collapse, coma, and even death.

FOXTAILS

A foxtail is a very common type of grass topped with a slender, spiky bristle. When this foxtail bristle gets caught in a dog's coat, the barbed end can pierce her skin, working its way farther and

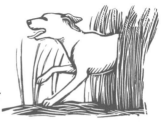

farther in as the dog moves. Foxtails are often found between a dog's toes, but the dog whose luck is not equal to her curiosity may have the painful misfortune of getting a foxtail up her nose. Foxtail is the most common type of imbedded foreign body to be taken out of dogs in this country. Obviously, dogs who spend a lot of time in the great outdoors—especially sporting or working dogs—are the most likely to encounter a foxtail. Of course, an embedded foxtail hurts, but of even more concern is the fact that bacteria are often carried into the wound with the spike—and into the body as far as the spike burrows. The resulting infections can be very serious, particularly those that occur in the chest.

WHAT TO DO ABOUT IT

The best strategy for foxtails is to avoid them completely. If you can't avoid them, be sure to check your dog thoroughly and keep her coat short during foxtail season. After outdoor adventures, carefully inspect your dog's entire coat, including between toes. If you find even the smallest sliver, remove it as soon as possible to prevent it from moving deeper into your dog's coat.

☏ WHEN TO CALL THE VET

If your dog has a foxtail and you can't remove it easily, take your pooch to the vet. Don't count on it to come out on its own. The longer you wait, the deeper it can go, so don't hesitate. The foxtail may have to be removed surgically, and the doctor may prescribe a course of antibiotics to curb any infection.

INSECT BITES AND STINGS

There are plenty of other tiny beasts to put the bite on your dog besides fleas. Ants, bees, wasps, flies, mosquitoes, and spiders may not be big, but their sting or bite can pack a painful wallop. Some dogs can even have an allergic reaction to a bee or wasp sting. Although an allergic reaction is more likely when the dog has been stung many times, it can still happen from just a single sting. An insect sting or bite produces those telltale small swollen areas; hot and swollen legs or face are often a sign of an allergic reaction.

Spiders are mostly inoffensive critters that like to hang out in places they're least likely to be disturbed: woodpiles, basements, old sheds, and the like. Most dogs meet up with spiders when they (the dogs) go nosing into those out-of-the-way places they (the spiders) love. That's why spider bites are most often found on a dog's face or front legs.

Some spiders, like the black widow and brown recluse, have potent venom. Within one to twelve hours, a dog bitten by a venomous spider may experience nausea, vomiting, chills, abdominal pain, difficulty breathing, and convulsions. Centipede stings may cause similar signs, as may the sting of a scorpion (not an insect, but a larger relative of the insects found in some parts of the country).

WHAT TO DO ABOUT IT

To soothe a simple insect sting, apply a baking powder paste. For a bee sting, look for the stinger—if you still see it in the skin, grasp the stinger at the skin line with tweezers and pull gently. Apply a cold compress to help bring the swelling down and reduce the pain.

WHEN TO CALL THE VET

Any sign of allergic reaction to an insect bite or sting, or any symptom of a venomous spider bite or scorpion sting should send you straight to your veterinarian. Any of these can rapidly develop into a life-threatening situation, and time is of the essence.

MANGE MITES

Everybody knows the term "mangy mutt," referring to a pooch who's seen better days. It conjures up the image of some poor broken-down mutt with a ratty, patchy coat. In fact, that's pretty much how dogs with mange really look. Mange is caused by an infestation of mange mites. It's Latin name, *Demodex canis*, gives rise to the other formal names for this condition: demodicosis or demodectic mange.

Most healthy dogs actually carry around a small population of Demodex mites. The trouble starts when there's a population explosion and the mites get out of control. Demodicosis can be localized, meaning it's found on only one area of the dog's body, or it can be generalized, spreading over the entire body. Localized demodicosis is more common, and it often clears up on its own. On the other hand, generalized demodicosis, which fortunately is pretty rare, requires the dog be dipped once or twice a week for six to eight weeks. The dog usually has to be shaved for the dip to be most effective.

Demodicosis is believed to be, at least in part, genetic, and dogs diagnosed with it should be neutered so they don't pass on the tendency. Breeds that tend to have more than their share of demodicosis are Afghan Hounds, American Pit Bull Terriers, American Staffordshire Terriers, Boston Terriers, Boxers, Bulldogs, Chihuahuas, Chinese Shar-Pei, Collies, Dalmatians, Dobermans, German Shepherd Dogs, Great Danes, Old English Sheepdogs, and Pugs.

Another type of mange mite, *Sarcoptes scabei* (var. *canis*), is the cause of sarcoptic mange—better known as scabies. This mite burrows into the skin's outermost layer and lays its egg. The eggs hatch, the larvae mature, and the emergent adult mites start the life cycle all over again. Scabies is highly contagious, and is one of the more common conditions that can be passed from dogs to people through direct contact.

WHAT TO DO ABOUT IT

The best treatment for mange is prevention. Regular brushing and baths will help remove scaly skin and scabs caused by mange and can help keep your dog mange-free. If your dog has been infested with mange mites, thoroughly wash his bedding or other sleeping areas. Do not try any other treatment at home until you take your dog to the vet.

Signs of localized demodicosis are patchy hair loss and scaly, reddened skin around the face or on the front legs. Generalized demodicosis has similar signs, but they are widespread and more severe, being especially likely to affect the feet. To diagnose demodicosis, your vet will gently scrape off some of the superficial layers of the dog's skin and examine them under the microscope to see if mites are present. If necessary, the vet will prescribe a dip and antibiotics to ward off any secondary infections caused by scratching. Unfortunately, demodicosis is persistent and recovery isn't guaranteed, especially in older dogs.

Signs of scabies are hair loss, small red bumps, and intense itching. Like demodectic mange, scabies is diagnosed through skin scrapings and treated with a weekly dip that your vet will prescribe. If your dog is diagnosed with scabies, you'll need to isolate her until her course of treatment is complete, and thoroughly clean everything she's been in contact with. Sarcoptic mange mites are extremely persistent, so other dogs in the household should also be treated, even if they don't show signs.

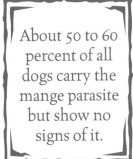

About 50 to 60 percent of all dogs carry the mange parasite but show no signs of it.

Porcupine Quills

You'd think one nose full of quills would be enough to put any dog off of her curiosity about porcupines. But some dogs never learn. If your dog is covered in quills, take her to the vet. But if she comes home with just a few prickles, you can try to remove them yourself.

What to Do About It

If your dog's snout gets converted into some porcupine's pincushion, get yourself some rubber gloves, a pair of needle-nose pliers, a dose of courage, and a strong-willed assistant to help you hold the dog. There's nothing pretty about the procedure, and there are no easy shortcuts: Just grasp each quill near the point of entry and pull straight out. Try not to break any quills; they'll be harder to remove, and any part of the quill left behind can encourage infection. Once you've removed the quills, apply a topical antiseptic to the affected area.

☎ When to Call the Vet

If you're leery about pulling out the quills yourself, bring your dog to your vet. If the dog has taken a large number of quills, or if the quills are imbedded in tricky or painful places (inside the dog's mouth, for instance) she will likely need sedation or even anesthesia.

Puncture Wounds

A puncture wound may be difficult to see because it's often covered with hair. The first sign may be a limp if it is on the leg or paw or slightly blood-tinged fur on other parts of the body. The most common location for puncture wounds is the bottom of the paw.

What to Do About It

If you notice your dog limping, examine her leg or paw for a small imbedded foreign object, such as a splinter, and remove it if possible. To do this, first clip the hair around the wound, then remove the object with tweezers or needle-nose pliers. Once you've removed the item, clean the wound with three-percent hydrogen peroxide. Do not bandage the wound, unless there is excessive bleeding. Puncture wounds are deceptive; they can be deeper than they look, often damaging muscle tissue and causing fluid to accumulate. Leaving the wound open to drain minimizes the risk of infection and swelling.

If you can't see or remove the foreign object, try drawing it out with a poultice of warm kaolin (a type of clay available at a drugstore or health food store). If this is unsuccessful, take the dog to your vet.

If the object is protruding from the dog, place sterile dressings around the point of entry, and take your dog to the vet immediately; do not try to remove the object. For excessive bleeding and chest wounds, bandage the wound tightly enough to seal it, and get your dog to the vet.

SCRAPES AND SCRATCHES

These abrasions damage the outer layers of skin. The most common cause of scrapes and scratches in dogs is other dogs—and even other neighborhood critters. Vigorous play, a miscalculation, or an out-and-out fight can result in wounds that need to be tended to right away.

WHAT TO DO ABOUT IT

Minor cuts and scratches should get the commonsense treatment: Wash well with soap and water, and let the area dry. Keep the area clean, and it should heal quickly. Don't try to prevent your dog from licking a scratch—that's Mother Nature's way of taking care of it. But do keep an eye on your dog to make sure she isn't overdoing it. She may require some kind of restraint to prevent mutilation of the wound.

☎ WHEN TO CALL THE VET

A more serious wound that won't stop bleeding needs immediate veterinary attention. Severe lacerations—ragged tears in the skin—need to be treated (and probably stitched) by your vet. The earlier this is done, the better chance of quick healing.

SORE FEET

A dog's foot pads are firm and thick, since they were designed by nature to endure tough surfaces. But durable as they are, a dog's paws are still susceptible to soreness, burns, and scrapes. Sore foot pads are a common aftereffect of a long day of hiking, walking on hot pavement in the summertime, or overdoing a play session due to a dog's natural exuberance.

What to Do About It

If your pet's paws are dog-tired, you can give her some relief with a thick paste of pine tar and Fuller's earth. Apply the mixture to the affected area to soothe and heal it. After an outdoor jaunt, always check your dog's paws for cuts and scratches. If your dog was running around in a muddy area, wash her paws with some soap and water, and dry her feet thoroughly.

☎ When to Call the Vet

Sore foot pads usually do not require a trip to the vet, unless you notice your dog is limping or you find a deep wound on her paw.

Sunburn

If your dog likes to sit in the sun—and what dog doesn't—you need to make sure she doesn't get too much of a good thing. Dogs are susceptible to sunburn, especially in areas where their fur is thinner, such as the tips of their ears or bridge of their noses. White- or light-coated dogs—like fair-skinned people—are especially prone to sunburn.

A sunburned dog shows the classic sign of reddened skin that peels and blisters. The result is sore and painful skin. Just as with people, excessive exposure to the sun can cause cancer in dogs.

What to Do About It

Protect your dog by limiting the amount of time she spends in the sun, using zinc oxide around the nose area, or applying sunscreen (careful with this—don't let her lick it off). There's even a sunscreen made specially for dogs, available at pet supply stores.

For sunburn pain, mist the affected area with a water bottle. The cool water will soothe some of the discomfort. A cold compress is another way to relieve the pain. Dampen a small towel and place it over the afflicted area. Rewet the towel when it starts to feel warm.

☎ WHEN TO CALL THE VET

A sunburn usually does not require a trip to the vet. However, if the skin is raw or broken or if your dog is visibly in pain, it's a good idea.

WORMS

COCCIDIA

Not really a worm but a one-celled microscopic organism, this parasite is not especially common in dogs, but it can strike young puppies, particularly when they're living in crowded conditions with lax sanitation. The disease is picked up through contaminated water, food, or surroundings. Coccidia produce eggs in the dog's intestinal tract, which are then passed into the environment in the stool. Coccidia can lie dormant, causing no symptoms, but they can be activated by some sort of stress. Once they swing into action, these little protozoans start doing their dirty work, causing diarrhea, weakness, lack of appetite, anemia, and dehydration. Your vet will probably treat Coccidia with sulfa drugs and antibiotics. Good hygiene is the key to containing and preventing Coccidia. Pick up the stool immediately, making sure there's no opportunity for food or water to be contaminated by it. If your dog is diagnosed with Coccidia, a thorough cleaning of her living area, using strong (but canine-safe) disinfectants or boiling water, is needed.

GIARDIA

This is another protozoal parasite—and it can affect dogs and people. Giardia is often waterborne, entering the water supply through contamination by wild animals, dogs, and people. Signs of Giardia infection are diarrhea, which may appear bloody or slimy, and sometimes a mild stomach upset. Your vet will treat Giardia with antiprotozoal drugs. Protect your dog from Giardia by not letting your dog drink from streams, rivers, or lakes, no matter how clean they may look.

HEARTWORM

Once restricted to the more hot and humid areas of the United States, and of most concern for dogs who spent a lot of time in the woods, heartworm is now prevalent in every part of the country.

The life cycle of the heartworm, *Dirofilaria immitis*, begins with the bite of a mosquito carrying heartworm larvae. The larvae enter the skin, going through several stages of development and eventually riding through the dog's bloodstream to the right side of the heart. Here they stay and become mature worms.

If not detected, the population of adult worms can grow, creating a mass that blocks blood flow, decreases the heart's efficiency, and eventually causes the right side of the heart to fail.

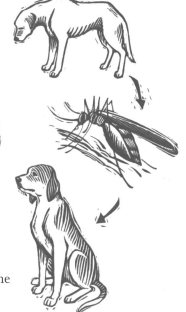

When the adult worms breed, they produce microfilaria. These are off-spring that enter the circulating blood and are small enough to be sucked up by a mosquito that bites the infected dog. Within 10 to 48 days, the microfilaria develop into infectious larvae. The next time the mosquito bites a dog, these heartworm larvae are passed along and the cycle begins all over again.

Dogs infested with heartworms may go for years without showing signs. When the heartworms eventually start to cause a dog trouble, an early sign may be a deep, soft cough that gets worse with exertion. As the cycle progresses, the dog becomes lethargic, loses weight, and sometimes coughs up blood. In the later stages of heartworm disease, the dog has trouble breathing, her chest bulges, and she develops congestive heart failure. Without treatment, she'll die.

Fortunately, a routine blood test can detect heartworm even before any signs appear. And heartworm can be easily prevented. Every dog should be tested for heartworm (your veterinarian can tell you when and how often). Most dogs will test negative, but your vet may still recommend a heartworm preventative. Diethylcarbamazine (DEC, which is sold under brand names such as Filaribits) kills the infective larvae. It must be given daily during mosquito season to make sure no larvae survive to mature into adult worms.

If a dog is diagnosed with heartworm, treatment depends on how far along things are. If there's heart failure or liver or kidney damage, those problems must be attended to first. The treatment for a full-blown case of heartworms is very stressful, and the dog must be in the best possible condition in order to survive it. Follow-up care is crucial, too. About six weeks after initial treatment, the recovering dog gets another drug to kill any microfilaria produced by the adult worms. A blood sample is checked to make sure all the microfilaria are gone. If it comes up positive, additional treatments are given until the dog is completely free of worms and microfilaria.

Hookworms

Hookworms are most often found in warm, humid areas of the country but can show up anywhere. These worms, the most common of which is known as *Ancylostoma caninum*, usually affect puppies, although adult dogs can have them, too. They're usually passed in the mother's milk or even through the skin and take up residence in the pup's small intestine. Once in the dog's belly, they hook onto the intestinal wall, sucking in tissue and blood. This causes one of the classic signs of hookworm infestation: dark, tarry, or bloody stool. In serious cases of hookworm disease, dogs suffer severe anemia.

Like most other intestinal worms, hookworms are diagnosed by examining a stool sample under a microscope. If hookworm eggs are found, your vet will probably prescribe medication to kill the adult worms. In areas of the country where hookworm is extremely common, a healthy dog with a mild case may not be treated, since she'll probably be reinfected quickly anyway. The best prevention for hookworm is being diligent in picking up after your dog. The longer an infected dog's stool sits, the more likely it is that any hookworm eggs will hatch out into larvae and find their way under your dog's skin.

ROUNDWORMS

Roundworms (*Toxocara canis*) are common in dogs, especially young puppies. Roundworm eggs are found in the soil, where they can survive for years. The life cycle of the roundworm seems unnecessarily difficult. The dog swallows the eggs from nosing around on the ground or picking something up in her mouth. The eggs hatch into larvae, ride through the bloodstream to the lungs and from there up the windpipe, where they're swallowed again, return to the intestine, and become mature adult worms. Roundworm larvae can also be passed from mother to puppies through the placenta (the pups are actually born with roundworms) or through the mother's milk.

Adult dogs can carry roundworms without much in the way of symptoms. But puppies with a load of them may vomit, have diarrhea, and lose weight. They have a noticeable pot belly (more than the usual "puppy tummy"), their coats are dull, and they don't thrive like other pups. Occasionally, a dog may pass some of the worms in her stool. These worms look like strands of wriggling white spaghetti.

Responsible breeders and shelters check their dogs and puppies for roundworms and other parasites, and give them the regimen of medication to knock out the uninvited guests. Puppies should have had a fecal exam and worming before they're old enough to be adopted, although follow-up doses of the medication may be needed. As with other types of worms, good sanitation is the key to prevention.

TAPEWORMS

Fleas are the most common carriers of tapeworm, although they can also be transmitted in small rodents or raw meat. So be careful in handling raw meat, and never feed your dog raw or undercooked meat or animal parts. If your dog has been treated for fleas, there's a good chance she's got tapeworms, too. The head—or scolex—of the tapeworm (the most common one in dogs is called *Dipylidium caninum*) hooks onto the intestine and begins producing a series of flat egg-filled segments resulting in a single worm with a length that can vary from a few inches to several feet. The most common way of diagnosing tapeworm is finding these segments—which look like grains of rice—in the dog's stool or clinging to the fur around the dog's anus.

Since the eggs are shed in the segments, a fecal exam can easily miss a tapeworm infestation. It's up to you to keep a close eye out for the segments themselves and for other possible signs, such as digestive trouble (usually seen in younger dogs with large infestations) and scooting. This type of behavior is defined by the dog dragging her rear end along the ground. Scooting can be a response to irritation from tapeworms, but it can also be a sign of an impacted anal gland—something your vet or groomer can remedy easily. Once tapeworm has been detected (or suspected), treatment is simple and effective. Prevention includes flea control and not feeding the dog raw or undercooked meat and animal products.

WHIPWORMS

Skinny little things with a bulge at one end, whipworms (*Trichuris vulpes*) are so named because their shape suggests a tiny whip. Dogs pick up whipworm eggs from the environment. The eggs hatch in a pooch's intestinal tract, where the worms latch onto the wall of the large intestine and start producing eggs all over again. Like other kinds of worms, whipworms are usually only noticeable in young or debilitated dogs. A heavy infestation may cause diarrhea, anemia, or weight loss.

Once again, treatment is a simple medication, usually repeated at least one more time to catch any recently hatched worms before they reinfect the dog. Since the eggs are shed in the infected dog's stool, prevention is a matter of common sense and common courtesy: Keep your dog away from the stools of other dogs, and pick up after your dog promptly. Regular fecal exams—twice a year is best—will catch a case of worms before it gets out of control.

ALTERNATIVE MEDICINE

Modern veterinary medicine has made many advances. New vaccinations, medications, diagnostic aids, and surgical techniques that were once undreamed of are realities, helping pets live longer, healthier lives. But some veterinarians are looking to the past to find successful treatments that rely on natural substances like herbs or homeopathic remedies, or physical manipulations like massage, chiropractic, or acupuncture. Alternative therapies have been used to treat skin problems, digestive upsets, and other conditions. Of course, an accurate diagnosis must be made before you begin any type of treatment, but many dogs can benefit from a skilled and sensible combination of traditional and alternative therapies.

Some veterinarians incorporate alternative methods into traditional practices, while others specialize in treatments like acupuncture or homeopathy. A veterinary degree is not required to practice some alternative therapies, although many states require that these therapies be administered to animals with veterinary supervision. With the proper training, however, both veterinarians and nonveterinarians can perform acupressure or massage on a pet. Here are some alternative therapies and their uses.

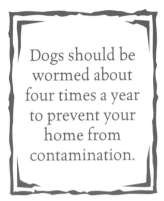

Dogs should be wormed about four times a year to prevent your home from contamination.

Acupuncture. The use of acupuncture and acupressure is thousands of years old. It was developed in ancient China and is based on the theory of energy flowing through a system of channels (called meridians) that flow through the body and are linked to certain internal organs. Disease is seen in large part as disharmony in this internal energy flow, and the purpose of acupuncture is to restore the balance. Acupuncturists may do this by using needles, finger pressure, heat sources, or other methods to manipulate certain specific points (or acupoints) along the meridians. Western scientific research is still at a loss to explain why acupuncture works. Some theories suggest that inserting the needles increases the body's production of endorphins (substances that make you feel better and more comfortable) and blocks the transmission of pain signals from the spinal cord to the brain.

When acupuncture was widely introduced in the West in the 1970s, the medical establishment didn't believe it worked. Since then, acupuncture has gradually gained respect as a viable treatment in many cases. In veterinary medicine, acupuncture has been used to treat allergies, arthritis, constipation, diabetes, kidney disorders, and liver disease.

With direction from a trained acupuncturist, you can provide home care for some conditions by manipulating your dog's meridians with finger pressure. Acupressure can be beneficial for dogs with arthritis, digestive disorders, and muscle strains.

Chiropractic. Developed in the 19th century, chiropractic is based on the idea that nerve energy flows through the spinal column. The energy becomes blocked if the spinal column is misaligned. Chiropractors manipulate the musculoskeletal system with fast, gentle motions (called adjustments) to restore normal movement or function to joints and surrounding tissues. As with acupuncture, we don't have a solid scientific explanation as to exactly why or how chiropractic works, but it has been used to treat a number of problems, from upset stomachs to arthritis.

Herbology. Herbs and flowers were probably among the first ways human beings treated sickness. We also know that animals will eat plants in response to certain illnesses. Today, some of our most widely used medications and treatments are plant-derived, including digitalis (foxglove), for certain heart conditions, and pyrethrins (chrysanthemums), a main ingredient in many flea-control products. The chemicals in herbal remedies have been found to strengthen the immune system, provide relief from pain, and calm the mind.

You may like the idea of using herbal remedies because they are natural, but like any other medication, medicinal herbs are dangerous if they're not used properly. They should be given only with veterinary supervision and in consultation with someone trained in the use of herbs. The safest, most effective way to use herbs at home is for treating external problems such as flea infestations or skin conditions. Before treating your dog with any herbal preparation, check with a qualified holistic veterinarian.

Homeopathy. Homeopathic medicine has been practiced for about 200 years and was originated by the German physician, Samuel Hahnemann. Through testing and observation, Hahnemann discovered that substances that produced certain reactions in healthy people—

such as the itchy, swollen bumps caused by bee venom—could stimulate a healing response in someone with an illness that had similar symptoms. Thus a homeopathic preparation of bee venom given to a person with a rash looking and feeling like bee stings alleviated the symptoms. This fundamental principal of homeopathy ("like cures like") was observed by the ancient Greeks and again in modern times with drugs like ritalin (a stimulant used to treat hyperactivity) and birth-control pills (the hormones that regulate fertility).

Before prescribing anything, a homeopathic veterinarian will question you about your dog's lifestyle, diet, and behavior. Once the environment is analyzed, the vet will prescribe a homeopathic remedy. In addition to homeopathic medications, the veterinarian may use tissue salts or flower essences to stimulate the body. Homeopathy is a true holistic healing modality: In addition to treating medical problems, homeopathic remedies are designed to take into account and treat related behavior and emotional issues.

Homeopathic remedies are prepared by successive dilutions and agitation of the original substance until there is little, if any, physical trace left. Because the active ingredients in common potencies of homeopathic remedies occur in such minute amounts, physical side effects are not an issue, making homeopathic remedies a safe, natural way to treat minor injuries and illnesses at home. Note: Homeopaths warn that using the wrong remedy may bring on a mild case of the symptoms that the remedy treats.

Common problems that respond to homeopathic remedies at home include minor stomach upset, bee stings or other insect bites, and minor injuries like cuts and scrapes. Other popular remedies include those that soothe the itching caused by flea bites and the anxiety caused by car travel or veterinary visits. Formulas for relieving the aches of arthritis; maintaining clean, healthy ears; and resolving mild cases of diarrhea are also available.

Massage. Massage does more than just feel good. A rubdown can help a dog recover more quickly from injury or illness, improve her flexibility and mobility, stimulate blood circulation, relieve muscle tension, and help keep her tissues supple. Depending on the strokes you use, a massage can energize or relax your dog.

Giving your dog a regular massage is a good way to become familiar with the feel of her body so you'll notice any unusual lumps, bumps, or other changes. A dog who gets massaged also gets used to being handled—something your vet and groomer will appreciate.

THE GOLDEN YEARS

Depending on their size and breed, dogs start to get old when they are six to eight years old. It's a good idea to take them in to the veterinarian for a special checkup at this age, just to make sure there aren't any serious problems lurking around. If you notice things early enough, treatment is likelier to be easier and less expensive. Some of the signs of aging you may see in your old dog include whitening of the muzzle, a thinning coat or dry fur, less energy than in younger years, a slower, stiffer gait, and cloudy eyes. Her hearing and sight might not be so good, and her teeth may start to look worn and yellow. But the one thing that won't diminish is the love she has for you.

QUALITY OF LIFE

Advances in veterinary medicine have dogs living longer than ever, but it's inevitable that the time will come when a beloved dog's days are at an end. It's one of the hardest things any pet owner has to do: Make the decision to say good-bye. How do you know it's time? In many cases, your dog will tell you. She won't feel like eating anymore, and she'll spend most of her time sleeping. It's a struggle for her to get up and go outside, and sometimes she doesn't make it. When she's not even interested in greeting you anymore, the time has probably come to give her a peaceful and dignified exit from life.

GIVING YOUR DOG A MASSAGE

Regular massage sends a clear message of love and trust between you and your dog. Light, long strokes using the full open palm and fingers is called effleurage. A deep rolling and kneading motion is petrissage. In-between is the light to medium pressure of fingertip massage. Fast, smooth strokes with your fingers in the direction the hair grows will energize your dog, while effleurage— moving from the nose to the tail—is a soothing way to end a massage.

Massage only for as long as your dog enjoys it. If you are massaging an old or anxious dog, use a light touch and move your fingers around the skin in big circles. This circular form of petting is sometimes more comfortable than other forms of touch, especially for dogs with arthritis. Don't massage dogs with cancer, broken bones, sprains, or ruptured vertebral disks.

Make no mistake about it. A dog is a special member of the family, and it's perfectly natural and normal for you to miss her and to grieve over her death. Don't let anybody tell you different. Express your grief to understanding friends and family. There are pet loss support groups and grief hotlines to help you handle your loss, too (see Chapter 10, "Where to Learn More"). Let the feeling run its course—it's the healthiest thing to do.

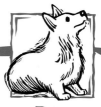

COMMON BEHAVIORAL PROBLEMS AND HOME REMEDIES

In most cases, behavior problems are really communication problems. When you stop to think about it, it's amazing humans and dogs can live together at all. Besides being totally different animals, we also see, hear, smell, taste, and feel the world very differently—and process it all through a very different brain.

Back when all dogs were wild, actions like chewing, scent-marking, and barking weren't an issue. Now that dogs are a regular part of human families, these natural behaviors can become problem behaviors. That means we have to shape a dog's natural behavior so it fits in with polite society—what we might call teaching a dog good manners.

Be Dominant but Not Domineering

Your relationship with your dog is based on dominance. Forget everything you know about dominance in people—it doesn't really apply to dogs. While it may seem a dominant dog is bigger, faster, stronger, or smarter than a subordinate dog, that's not always the case. And once a dominance relationship is established between two adult dogs, the subordinate dog doesn't think about how he can get ahead. It's the consistency of the relationship that keeps the peace and keeps dogs happy.

Dominance is both the glue and the lubricant of canine society—a unit of two or more dogs known as the pack. Even if there's just you and your dog in your home, your dog sees that as his pack. One of you has to be the top dog, and if it isn't you, he'll step into the role. That's the beauty of the human-canine relationship. If you establish dominance, you can control a dog who not only outweighs you but could eat you for lunch, yet would never even consider doing it.

So it should be clear that dominance is not so much a physical thing in dogs as it is a state of mind. A dominant dog is not a bully—a dominant dog is a peacekeeper. Sometimes he has to discipline subordinate dogs, but he can also control them simply by his presence, a look, or a single sound of his voice. That's how obedience training works in establishing dominance. If you can get your dog to stop doing something you don't want him to do by approaching him, looking at him, or giving a single command, you are the top dog. But with authority comes responsibility. You have to be certain you are communicating dominance consistently and in a way your dog understands.

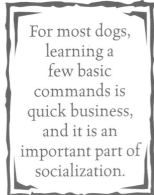

For most dogs, learning a few basic commands is quick business, and it is an important part of socialization.

Several of the behavior problems in this chapter are related to dominance. Establishing a good dominance relationship with your dog is the best preventative—and the best cure.

AGGRESSION

Aggression is probably the most common reason an otherwise healthy dog is euthanized (put to sleep). We sometimes forget dogs are predators and can inflict serious and even fatal wounds. A truly aggressive dog is terrifying—and rightfully so.

You need to understand if your dog is really displaying aggression. The word aggression has a specific meaning in the field of animal behavior. It's also relative: What would be aggressive to us may be perfectly ordinary to a dog. A good example is play. A child who chased another child across a field, bit him on the back of the neck, and pulled him down to the ground at a dead run would be acting pretty aggressively. However, to a pair of playing dogs, that's an accurate description of a good time. Play is often viewed as practice for real-life skills, so it's not unusual to see stalking, chasing, hunting, and even killing behaviors as part of normal dog play.

So how can you tell? Usually by the look and sound. Does the dog have a play face (wide-open eyes and relaxed-open jaws, like a big, toothy grin)? Is the behavior accompanied by furious or loud snarling and barking? Or is it play-growls and happy yips? A surefire sign is if the roles reverse: If there's a chase on and suddenly the chasing dog changes direction and is being pursued, you can bet it's play.

There are several reasons why your dog may display aggressive behavior. Here are the types of aggression.

Defensive. Here's a classic scenario for defensive aggression: The dog does something wrong; the owner catches the dog and scolds him; the dog then retreats under the bed; the owner reaches under the bed to pull the dog out and reprimand him for the misdeed; and the dog bites the owner.

Any dog will bite when he feels threatened. In this case, the dog gave ground and made himself "invisible," which is submissive behavior in dog society. The only reason the dog could think of to explain why the owner was still pursuing him after he had submitted to the owner's dominance was the owner intended to do him harm. So the dog protected himself. The best thing to do if your dog retreats is to just leave him alone.

Territorial. Territorial aggression is one of the reasons we like living with dogs. They will defend their territory—which can include our home, our possessions, their food, and us—against all comers. Without territorial aggression, there would be no watchdogs.

But territorial aggression can get out of hand. It can pop up in things as minor as jumping up, as frustrating as marking territory, or as serious as biting. Again, a good dominance relationship with your dog is crucial. If you're the dominant dog, he'll feel secure when you feel secure—and won't defend territory against friendly visitors, meter readers, and letter carriers—but will still defend you and your home when the need arises.

Agonistic (pain-related). A sick or injured dog knows he is vulnerable. The same is true for an aging dog, whose senses have dulled, reactions have slowed, and mobility has decreased. Even ordinary situations can make a vulnerable dog feel the need to lash out in his own defense.

Sometimes the dog's pain is obvious, and you can be ready for possible aggression. Other times, however, it's not so easy to tell until it's too late. If you're petting or playing with your dog as usual, for example, and he suddenly growls or snaps at you, you should suspect something hurts and call the vet right away. Arthritis is a common cause for this type of behavior.

Reproductive. This one probably needs no explanation. If there's a female dog in heat anywhere in the known universe, unneutered male dogs know it and will try to get through everything—including each other—to reach her. The drive to reproduce can trigger fighting with other dogs and even uncharacteristic aggression toward family members.

The surefire solution for this type of aggression is obvious but important: You must neuter or spay your dog, preferably before the age of six months.

☎ When to Call the Vet

Aggressive behavior isn't something that can be ignored or laughed off. Your dog's life depends on it. If your dog is launching serious attacks, especially without warning or provocation, get him in for a thorough veterinary exam as soon as possible. Your vet can help you determine a course of treatment or refer you to a competent behaviorist. Though aggression can sometimes be related to a physical problem, such as a brain tumor, encephalitis (infections of the brain), lead poisoning, low blood sugar, or liver disease, it is usually a behavioral problem. If your dog shows any form of aggressive behavior, call your vet or an animal behavioral specialist immediately.

Biting

Each year, anywhere from half a million to one million dog-bite injuries are reported. The most likely victims of dog bites are children under 12 years old (accounting for about 60 percent of the total), and

BITE-PROOFING: AVOIDING BITES FROM STRAYS AND OTHER DOGS

If you're facing a dog who's exhibiting threatening behavior, how you respond (or don't respond) can make the difference between getting away safely and getting bitten. Any dog can bite, so don't assume the dog you know who's growling and staring won't hurt you. Similarly, an unfamiliar dog who isn't showing threatening behavior should not be assumed to be friendly. Since children are at highest risk for dog bites, teach youngsters in the family these basic techniques—and practice them yourself.

The most important rule to remember is: Never approach any strange dog. If the dog approaches you, don't run. Stand perfectly still (tell young children to stand like a tree), with your fists folded underneath your chin and your elbows close to your body. Keep your legs together and look straight ahead, not at the dog. (Remember, staring is a threat gesture.) If the dog approaches you while you're on the ground, roll onto your stomach with your legs together, fists folded behind your neck, and forearms covering your ears (tell kids to act like a log). Remain still until the dog goes away.

the top five perpetrators are Chow Chows, Rottweilers, German Shepherd Dogs, Cocker Spaniels, and Dalmatians. In the general dog population, unneutered male dogs are the most likely to bite. In other words, keeping an unneutered male Chow in a home with a two-year-old, a five-year-old, and twin eight-year-olds will probably guarantee you'll take at least one bite-motivated trip to the emergency room. This doesn't mean you should never have bite-prone breeds or that you must wait until the kids are in high school before getting a dog. It does mean you need to have a better understanding of why and when dogs bite, and take steps with your dog and your family to bite-proof your household.

In at least half of all reported dog-bite cases, the bites were provoked by the victim—although often unintentionally. Dogs usually give clear signals they're ready to bite—clear, at least, to other dogs and to people who know how to recognize them. The most common dog-bite scenario involves a person or young child who misses the dog's warning sign and gets within range. The other common cause of bites is miscommunication. Perhaps the best known example is the encounter between a child and a stray dog: Frightened by the sudden appearance of a large and unfamiliar pooch, the child instinctively screams and runs away. This triggers the dog's chase reflex or is misinterpreted as play behavior. Either way, the only way the dog has of catching the child is with his mouth.

Classic canine body language that signals a dog's readiness to bite includes staring, bared teeth, growling, stiff-legged stance (it almost looks like the dog is standing on the tips of his toes), raised hackles (the fur on his shoulders, back, and rump), and a wagging tail with a stiff, rapid movement. Usually, your final warning is a more intense stare and deeper growling. When the dog's head is lowered and the ears go back against his head, you can expect the next thing you hear to be the sound of his teeth snapping together on whatever of yours he can get a hold of. Of course, it doesn't have to come to that. A wise person will back off well before it gets to this point.

☎ WHEN TO CALL A BEHAVIORIST

If the potentially threatening dog you encounter is your own, you may need professional help. Dogs may bite out of fear, defense, pain, or to protect territory—all reasons too subtle for you to detect without knowing what to look for. A trained behaviorist can help you pin down the reason for your dog's biting as well as develop a strategy to change the behavior. This might be as simple as giving the dog more exercise; socializing with people and other dogs; or teaching all family members to leave the dog alone while he's eating, sleeping, or hiding. However, it may involve a more extensive overhaul of your relationship with your dog.

CHASING CARS

"I'm not so concerned about Old Blue chasing cars," says my old pal, Hoke Mitchell. "It's when he brings 'em home and buries 'em in the yard that I start to get worried."

Hoke's dusty jokes aside, car chasing is a problem for some dogs. Some car chasers are just answering the instinctive call to the hunt: Anything that moves can serve as the prey. Others may be acting on territorial instincts, driving away (no pun intended) the motorized intruder from their turf. Still others—usually herding breeds or mutts with strong herding instincts—are trying to get those wayward cars back into the "flock." Basically, any dog will be inclined to give chase to a moving object—a tossed stick or ball, a passing cat or squirrel—but the trick is to teach him when chasing is okay: Fetching sticks and catching a ball are fine; trying to fetch the neighbor's cat and catch passing cars aren't.

First, try to figure out why your dog chases cars. Out here in the country where things are more spread out and neighbors might live up to a mile apart, letter carriers deliver the mail in little Jeeps. A car-chasing dog might view the daily arrival of this red-white-and-blue thing at the end of the access road as a regular attempt to crash his gate. Once the motive for the dog's chasing is understood, the solution may be as easy as introducing the dog to his nemesis. A few friendly encounters—perhaps punctuated by a favorite game or treat—and the threat evaporates, as does the car chasing.

Predatory chasing can often be corrected using a leash or a distraction (such as an unpleasant noise) to interrupt the start of the chase. When the dog turns his attention away from the chase, reinforce the behavior with praise (and an occasional treat). Of course, the surefire method to keep your dog from chasing cars is to keep him safely fenced or leashed.

Try giving the dog who sees cars as wayward sheep something more constructive to do with his herding instincts. Give him plenty of exercise, including several long walks or runs each day, or play running and jumping games with a frisbee. These dogs are good candidates for organized sports like flyball and agility training, too. If you have a herding dog (like a Collie or Sheltie), the best thing to do is train him for herding trials—after all, it's what they were born and bred to do! Again, this is something you should consider before you adopt a dog from a herding breed. It takes a lot of time to keep a dog like this busy, but you'll both be happier you made the investment.

☎ WHEN TO CALL THE VET

This type of behavior usually doesn't require any veterinary attention.

CHEWING

A dog's mouth is the canine equivalent of our hands; it's what dogs use to pick up and examine things, evaluate their potential use, and transport them from one place to another. Chewing lets a dog know what something feels like, how it tastes, and whether it's good to eat. It's a natural part of dog behavior: You can no more train a dog to stop chewing completely than you can train him to stop breathing. Chewing is also an important part of the pup's development. Just like babies, puppies chew in part to soothe sore gums during teething. It can take up to a year for a pup's adult teeth to come in, so this is another instance where you'll need lots of patience to teach your dog what he can chew and what he can't.

Naturally, your dog will be attracted to anything with your scent on it, so be sure to put away shoes, socks, and other items you've handled that you don't want destroyed. In fact, getting a puppy is terrific incentive to get everyone in your household to pick up clothes, shoes, and toys—if you don't, the odds are they'll be gnawed into oblivion. It won't take too many instances of a favorite item getting shredded before even the most careless family member is putting things away. Never give a dog old shoes or clothing to chew on. Shoes especially will retain your scent. In fact, never give your dog anything as a chew toy that is the same as something you don't want him to chew; he won't be able to tell the difference between the old boot you gave him to gnaw and your new hiking boots.

Make those toys you want your dog to chew (and he should have a number of them) as appealing as possible. If he seems to be going exclusively for things with your scent on them, put chew toys in the laundry hamper for a day or two before giving them to your dog. Rubbing something tasty on the outside of rubber balls or other toys or stuffing treats inside of hollow toys can encourage the dog to select those items to chew on his own. In general, be sure you're giving him the message clearly from the beginning. Give him the appropriate toys to chew, and praise him for chewing them. Always keep a chew toy within reach (even carry one with you). If you see your dog working on something you don't want him to chew, quickly remove the item and replace it with the toy, then immediately praise him for chewing the correct item. There a million things in your home you don't want him to chew; it's much easier to teach him to recognize the handful of items he *can* chew.

If you want to give your dog bones to chew on, stick to large knuckle-bones or thigh bones. Before you hand them out, sterilize bones by boiling them for half an hour. Never give small bones or bones that could splinter easily, such as chicken or turkey bones.

Some dogs remain very active chewers all their lives. Destructive chewing is especially common in dogs who spend a lot of time alone, since it's a way of working off boredom or anxiety. "Home alone" dogs need to have lots of different toys, which should be rotated to keep things interesting. When you're home with the dog, be sure he gets lots of exercise and quality time with you.

☎ WHEN TO CALL THE VET

As with any behavior problem, have your vet take a look at your dog before you start any corrections. On occasion, a destructive chewer is signaling his teeth or gums are bothering him. If there's a physical cause for the behavior, no amount of training or correction will change it.

COPROPHAGY (EATING STOOL)

Dogs will eat just about anything, including their own feces or that of other animals. As disgusting as this sounds, it's common enough to get a fancy medical name: coprophagy, from the Greek *kopros* (dung) and *phagos* (one who eats).

Yes, it's an unpleasant topic. But you have to realize sometimes coprophagy is a natural and normal act. Newborn puppies haven't yet learned to eliminate on their own, so the mother dog licks them to stimulate urination and defecation, and then licks them again to clean them up. In other circumstances, nature will prevent all that waste from . . . well, going to waste. For instance, cats need a higher percentage of fat in their diets than dogs, which means a higher level of waste fat in their stool. Anyone who has dogs and cats knows the pooch will have his nose in the litter box, searching out the leftover nutrient in "kitty chocolates."

When adult dogs eat their own stool, though, it's a different story. Usually, it's a sign of loneliness or boredom, although on occasion, miscues in housebreaking will result in the dog eating stool because

How to Prevent Chewing

Of course, the most important part of prevention for chewing is common sense: Keep everything you don't want chewed out of your dog's reach, or keep your dog out of areas where nonchewable things can be easily found. Dogs who chew only when left alone can be put into their kennels or crates. (Never use the crate as punishment. The crate should be thought of as your dog's den—a safe and happy place.)

Since you can't put things like the sofa or dining room table on a high shelf, you'll have to resort to other methods. Some trainers recommend applying a mixture of cayenne pepper in petroleum jelly or some other unpleasant-tasting substance to furniture legs and other potential chewing zones. (Test the substance on an inconspicuous spot first to make sure it won't damage the finish.) Upholstery can be protected by putting double-sided tape (or a flattened loop of masking tape, sticky side out) on items such as furniture skirting, curtains, and bedspread hems. If the tacky feel doesn't dissuade your dog from chewing, you can try dusting the outside with a non-toxic, unpleasant-tasting substance such as cayenne pepper.

Corrections for chewing inappropriate items should only be made when you catch your dog in the act. Never reprimand a dog after the fact. No matter how much you think he looks like he knows he's been bad, he's really only reacting to you and your anger. Instead, when you catch him chewing something you don't want him to, quickly take away the incorrect item (you can also interrupt the unwanted chewing with a shaker can or other distraction for emphasis), immediately substitute it with a chew toy, and then praise him lavishly.

he's learned the presence of stool sometimes gets him punished. Actually, coprophagy doesn't present any problem for dogs, with the possible exception of eating stool containing parasite eggs. It is a major aesthetic problem for the owner, however, who must witness it and whose face the dog then tries to lick. You can try to break the habit by relieving the dog's boredom or loneliness: Give him more attention and exercise, rotate his toys so he doesn't have to play with the same old thing all the time, and feed him more than once a day so he has something to look forward to.

Prevention is the only sure cure. Pick up after your dog right away, or muzzle a coprophagic dog when walking in public areas. Set up cat litter boxes where Rex can't get his nose into them—or simply keep them clean of stool by scooping several times a day, especially before and after feline mealtimes.

When to Call the Vet

As soon as you notice this behavior, make a trip to the vet—there may be a physical cause for a dog's coprophagy. A bellyful of worms or other parasites could rob Rex's body of vital nutrients, and he might be eating whatever he can find to try and make up for it. There might also be a nutritional deficiency in his diet. Adding brewer's yeast to his food will boost his intake of B-vitamins. Pumpkin or raw carrot will add fiber to his diet and help him feel full. In some cases, solving the problem is as simple as switching Rex over to a food with more fat, fiber, or protein. Your vet can recommend a brand better suited to Rex's dietary needs.

Digging

Digging is another natural behavior in dogs. They do it for lots of reasons. Terriers, for example, do it simply because they've been bred to do it for countless generations—part of their original job of digging out burrows and going in after varmints like rats and badgers.

Other dogs dig to fix themselves a place to sleep, to stash some food, to make a secure hiding place, or out of pure boredom. And some do it just because it's fun.

If your dog has started excavating your yard or digging holes in your love seat, try to figure out his motive. Is he bored and trying to while away the hours doing a little relandscaping? Is he trying to beat the heat by making a bed in the cool earth? Is he an unneutered male trying to get under the fence and after that female on the next street? Or maybe he's burying bones or other treats to enjoy later on? Once you think you have a handle on his reason for digging, you can take steps to change the behavior.

Now, if your dog is one of those who's been bred to dig, you've got a tough row to hoe. You're never going to get him to quit, so you're going to need to give him the opportunity to dig where it's okay. Try giving him his own plot of dirt or a sandpit (fewer muddy tracks) to dig in. Encourage him to dig there, and praise him when he does. Keep the area appealing with lots of toys and treats. If he digs because he's trying to find a cooler place to lie down, simply provide more shade in that spot or move him to a place where he can be more comfortable—under a tree or in the house, for instance. The dog who's trying to escape might be a little more difficult to deal with. Some people have gone so far as to put concrete or wire beneath their fences to keep

Nordic breeds such as the Samoyed enjoy digging, even though it is unlikely that today's incarnation would need to scrape out a cozy nest in the snow the way their ancestors did.

digging dogs in. Neutering or spaying takes away a major motive for escape. Other dogs feel anxious or threatened out in the open for long periods of time. Sometimes, just providing shelter—access to a garage, shed, or doghouse—is enough to put an end to the great escape.

Again, use distraction techniques when you catch your dog in the act of digging where you don't want him to. As soon as he stops, praise him, play a favorite game, give him a toy, or take him to his designated digging area. Never correct a dog for digging after the fact. This only confuses him, making him anxious and more likely to dig!

☎ WHEN TO CALL THE VET

Digging behavior usually doesn't require any veterinary attention.

FIGHTING

Dogs get into scrapes with other dogs as a way of figuring out who's dominant to whom in canine society, to defend territory (including mating rights), out of fear, to protect their food, and sometimes as a defensive "first strike" when they encounter a dog who has attacked them in the past. A neutered or spayed dog who has spent his formative early weeks of life with his mom and litter-mates and has had plenty of socialization since—with other dogs and people, too—has the best chance staying out of fights. Of course, all that is water under the bridge once you have an adult dog who is a fighter. You might never be able to teach this dog to enjoy being around his fellow canines, but you can take steps to keep the situation under control.

Your reaction determines how your dog will react to other dogs. If you anticipate trouble when you see other dogs headed your way, your dog will pick up on your uneasiness and immediately perceive the approaching dog as a threat. Keep a loose lead, keep moving, and keep up a happy stream of conversation. Your dog needs to learn to view the approach of other dogs as normal, not negative.

TALES FROM THE COUNTRY VET:
MIXED BREED, MIXED INSTINCTS

I believe you get the best of all the traits in the breeds that
make up a mutt. Of course, you can't always tell what breeds
those are just by looking—and that can sometimes be a
problem. Take this client of mine who picked up a stray
mixed-breed female, just under a year old. Elsa was one of the
happiest dogs I've ever seen, but she had some horrible
habits. Within six months, this pooch had ripped apart a sofa
and two chairs, chewed up a tape player and a portable telephone, destroyed an area rug in the dining room, and peed
on just about every square inch of floor in the house.

"Sounds to me like frustrated instincts," I told her desperate
owner. "Watch her carefully when you have her outside, and
I'll bet she'll tell you what's bothering her."

A week later, the owner called back. "I didn't really believe
you at first, Doc," he said, "but you were right! First I took
Elsa down to run along the lake and she went immediately to
the shore and dug a hole in the sand. Then she practically
dove into the water. Finally, on our way back through the
park, we passed some kids playing soccer—and she goes
dashing off, barking and nipping at their heels, trying to herd
them all together!"

With regular trips to the beach to dig and swim, Elsa's terrier
and retriever instincts were satisfied. With regular games of
chase, her herding instincts were satisfied. With the addition
of obedience training and a dog crate, all the destructive and
housebreaking problems quickly disappeared.

Every dog, especially one who's prone to fighting, should be obedience trained. When another dog approaches, require your dog to go through an obedience routine or perform some other activity to take his attention off the other dog and focus it on you. If he starts growling or barking at the new arrival, you can now legitimately correct him for failing to respond to commands, not because of the approach of another dog.

Reproduction is a driving force behind territorial and aggressive fighting. Neutering a male dog is an absolute must for controlling and correcting fighting. Female dogs can be aggressive, too, and spaying is just as important. In fact, neutering and spaying have significant, long-range health and behavior benefits for all dogs.

☎ WHEN TO CALL A BEHAVIORIST

All dogs are not created equal, especially when it comes to dominance. If there's fighting between two dogs in your own household, they may be trying to figure out who answers to whom. A behaviorist can help you understand what's going on and offer advice on how to solve the problem. Remember, to a dog, being dominant or subordinate is a perfectly normal and natural thing. Don't make the mistake of thinking your dogs must treat each other as equals.

FOOD GUARDING

Instinct tells a dog to protect his food. However, it's important for you to have complete control over what goes into your dog's mouth. Part of this is for safety. If your dog starts to pick up something dangerous or deadly, such as rat poison, you need to be able to get it away from him without losing your fingers. However, access to food is also a dominance issue: When your dog responds by taking his food or dropping things out of his mouth on command, he is recognizing you as the dominant dog. Food guarding is a frequent trigger for dog bites, too. Therefore, the sooner you can establish that you and other family members are the ultimate authority when it comes to meals, the better off you'll be.

If your food guarder is still a puppy, you need to let him know everything he gets comes through you: food, toys, even petting. Tell your puppy to sit or lie down before you feed him, and make him wait until you give the release word, such as okay or take it, before he starts to chow down. If he comes up and nudges you for attention, use the same tactic to make it your initiation. He should also learn it's okay for you to touch him while he eats, so give him a pat when you put down his dish, and make it a habit to add a little food to his bowl while he's eating. This way, when you are near his food dish, it is always a happy occasion.

Location means everything when you feed your dog. If he's off in a corner, he may feel more possessive than if he were eating in a more spacious area with room to move around. Practice giving him food and taking it away. To do this, give your dog very small portions at a time. Each time he finishes a serving, take his dish away and refill it with another small amount until all his food is gone. As you take away and replace the dish, praise him for being a good dog. Once he's responding well to having his dish removed and replaced, move on to the next step: adding the food to his dish while it's still in front of him. Let him eat some of the food while you're off doing something else, then walk up and add something special to the dish, such as a piece of hot dog or a liver treat.

Let's get one thing clear, though: All this is so you have the ability to control what goes into your dog's mouth. Practice these techniques now and then so you can maintain your dominance relationship with your dog. The most important thing to remember is not to pester your dog while he's eating. Since most of Rover's meals should be in peace, teach all household members—especially children—that he is to be left alone at mealtime.

GUARDING OTHER POSSESSIONS

Lisa is a working single mom with two young children, ages 4 and 7. She got their dog, Hugo, from the pound as a companion for her kids and protection for the house. Hugo is a sweet-natured dog, excellent with the kids. However, he often growls and bares his teeth at them when he has a toy. "I don't get it," Lisa told the behaviorist. "My kids can just walk into the room where he's sitting with his toys and he growls. He even brings a ball for them to throw, chases it, and then snarls at them when he brings it back!"

A dog who's possessive about possessions is making a statement—you just need to make sure you're understanding it. In Lisa's case, part of the problem was a miscue on playing. Hugo loved to play fetch, but after several rounds of running down a tennis ball, he just wanted to lay down and chew. Unfortunately, the children thought his flopping on the ground a few feet away was part of the game and would take the ball away and throw it again. Hugo learned the only way he could end the game was to act threatening.

In other cases, it's more a matter of dominance. Using the same techniques as for food guarding can be effective, but owners often need to be assertive in other ways, too. Keeping the dog on a leash—even in the house—sends a clear message you're in control and everything is fine. Obedience-train your dog, and when he starts guarding a toy, issue a command, changing the focus from the toy to the behavior required. Praise him when he responds to the command (even if you had to correct him or use the leash to get him to do it). As part of his obedience training, every dog should have a command to stop him from picking something up or drop something already in his mouth. (Variations of this command are "Drop it!," "Leave it!," "Don't touch!," and "Out!")

If a particular kind of toy causes the green-eyed monster to visit your dog, dump it. Bones are especially likely to turn even the nicest dogs into jealous, possessive brutes. If your dog can't handle them—or certain other toys—don't give them to your dog. Don't forget to lavish your dog with praise when he does something right. Any time your dog turns away from a toy to respond to a command or lets you take something away, don't hesitate to tell him what a great dog he is. The amount of praise you give should always outweigh the number of corrections you make.

When to Call a Behaviorist

If guarding behavior becomes a recurring problem for your dog, an animal behaviorist can recommend the proper course of treatment. Once a remedy has been established, make sure all household members learn how to approach this problem.

Jumping Up

A young associate in a Chicago law firm showed up at work one morning with a cast on his arm and a medical collar on his neck. His co-workers couldn't resist the lawyer jokes: "Ambulance stop unexpectedly?" "Do you need a good attorney?" The fellow looked sheepish. "Nope—actually, my Great Pyrenees 'Dino-ed' me," he said, making reference to Fred Flintstone's overly exuberant dinosaur "dog."

Whether it's a body slam from a bubbly big breed or the frenzied hind-leg ballet of a toy pooch, jumping up is a universal trait—and problem—in our canine companions. There's no doubt this behavior is cute in puppyhood, but as a puppy grows—especially if he's a big dog—what was once cute can be downright dangerous. You may not mind the full-contact greeting, but the first time your two-year-old niece or 87-year-old aunt gets decked coming in the front door, you'll think very differently.

In fact, even though jumping up can be solicitous, friendly behavior, it is more often a dominance thing. Especially in adult dogs, a subordinate would never think of putting his front paws on the body of a

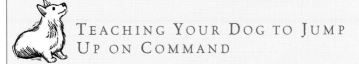

TEACHING YOUR DOG TO JUMP UP ON COMMAND

If you want to teach your dog to jump up only on command, be sure your dog first knows when not to jump up. Wear clothes you don't mind getting dirty or torn, and make sure your dog's nails are trimmed and filed. (It might be a good idea to brush his teeth, too!) Pat your chest and say, "Up!" When you want the dog to get down, step back and say, "Off!" (Don't use the word down or you will confuse him when you try to teach the down command.)

Always use the chest pat and the word up to let your dog know it's okay to greet you this way. If he tries to jump up on you or anyone else without an invitation, firmly tell him, "Off," and then ignore him. Dogs are smart, and Bruno will get the message that he is only allowed this behavior when you say it's okay. Be sure your friends and family follow this routine, too, or Bruno will be one confused dog. Dogs like rules, and they like everyone to follow the same rules.

dominant dog. So the excited, shot-from-a-cannon greeting that makes you feel good may actually be your dog saying, "You came back! Okay. Just remember I'm the top dog here." You can respond on two fronts: Teach your dog spontaneous jumping up is not acceptable, and train him to jump up on command when you say it's okay.

To curb his overly physical greeting, act as relaxed and laid-back as you'd like him to be. When you come home, don't run into the house, calling excitedly for your pup. Instead, make his greeting part of a routine rather than a special event. Walk in the door, hang up your coat and keys, and then greet the dog calmly, away from the front door. If Bruno tries to jump up, step aside and don't pay any attention to him. Like kids, dogs love to be noticed, whether it's for good behavior or bad. Yelling at your dog or kneeing him in the chest will only excite him more, so avoid any kind of verbal or physical reinforcement of his jumping. Once your dog learns you don't want him to jump on you, teach him to sit when you come home. If you reward the sit with a treat or praise, your dog will soon learn good things come to he who sits and waits.

☎ WHEN TO CALL THE VET

This type of behavior usually doesn't require any veterinary attention.

MARKING TERRITORY

We can't even imagine how the world smells to a dog. A dog's sniffer is an incredibly fine-tuned, delicate instrument compared to our own sniffer. It makes sense, then, that scent-marking—spraying urine on places and objects to mark territory and claim ownership—is an important part of canine communication. The chemical scent-messages in a dog's urine tell other dogs just about everything they need to know: where the marking dog hangs out, how long it's been since he's been around, and (in the case of a female) sexual receptivity. A dog who's nervous because he's home alone may mark furniture or walls to reassure himself everything is alright. Scent-marking can also be a way of asserting dominance, which is why some dogs will lift their legs on other dogs or even people.

Scent-marking is a perfectly normal and natural behavior that is instinctive in your dog. The idea is to let your dog know it is only to be done at specific places and times and not on your living room rug, bathroom floor, or bedspread. Once again, your dominance relationship with your dog can make all the difference. Obedience-train your dog in a positive and humane way, and run him through his commands regularly. This not only clarifies your dominance, it gives a dog who gets bored, lonely, or anxious during the day something to look forward to. Make him work for food, toys, play, and petting. If he wants one of those, have him respond to a command or two first.

Always walk through doors before he does, and don't let him jump up on you or get on the furniture, especially your bed. In canine society, you usually only get to jump on or lay next to an equal or subordinate dog. Neutering, especially before the dog is one year old, is another good preventative. Your dog will still be protective of home and family, but he won't have a hormone-driven desire to stake out reproductive territory.

Spraying due to separation anxiety is another matter. Your best bet here is to slowly get your dog used to being home by himself. Start with something simple, like leaving him alone in a room for just a minute or two and then returning. Then leave the house, returning after a few minutes. Each time you practice this, stay away for just a little bit longer. Once your dog learns you always come back, he'll be more comfortable staying by himself. Confining him to a crate can also help him feel more secure.

To deter your dog from spraying furniture, attach a piece of aluminum foil to the area where your dog likes to spray. The next time he does it, the urine hitting the foil will make a noise and may also splash back on him.

Finally, don't confuse scent-marking with an ordinary housebreaking problem. A large puddle of urine on the kitchen floor or near the back door is probably a sign the dog needed to get outside while you were gone—not a display of dominance!

☎ WHEN TO CALL THE VET

As with any behavior problem, have your vet take a look at your dog before you start any corrections. If there's a physical cause for the behavior, no amount of training or correction will change it.

Pulling on the Leash

Try this simple experiment. With your dog standing calmly in front of you, gently push backward on his chest or the front of his neck. What happens? Most dogs will lean into the pressure. This natural response has been bred to a science in sled dogs such as the Siberian Husky and in breeds who were originally also used as draft animals, including the Newfoundland Retriever. You've got absolutely no chance of controlling one of these born-to-pull dogs with brute strength.

We've all seen even tiny dogs straining at the end of the leash, bodies close to the ground, tongues lolling, breathing with a loud, choking rasp. The same instinct is at work. The trick is to teach your dog how to walk nicely on a leash from the very beginning. You don't have to expect him to walk perfectly on heel, but he should be able to stay with you without pulling, and he should make all the starts, stops, and turns that you do. If you use a jewel-link training collar (don't think of it as a choke collar—that's not how you should use it), any time the dog begins to pull, give a quick snap and release on the leash and tell him, "Heel" or "Slow" (whichever word you choose, be consistent). When he backs off, praise him.

Another alternative is a head collar—a device similar to a horse halter. Marketed under the name Gentle Leader or Promise, it's widely available through veterinarians and trainers. The collar loops around the dog's muzzle and behind his ears, with the leash snapping on under his chin. Since you control his head with the head collar, all the rest of him can't help but follow. Instead of hitting the end of the leash, feeling the pressure on his neck, and instinctively pulling harder, a dog in a head collar ends up getting his nose turned back toward you, slowing him down immediately. A retractable leash can also help keep pulling under control. Because it expands and contracts with the dog's movement, the dog has nothing to pull against. The brake allows you to control where the dog walks.

INTRODUCING DOGS AND KIDS

Dogs and kids just seem to go together—both are as rambunctious as can be. When I became a father, I made sure I taught my children to respect our dogs and treat them kindly. You need to do the same if you want your kids to enjoy the magical friendship that can exist only between a dog and a child.

Here are some basic rules your children should know about getting along with dogs. Most of them are simply a matter of understanding canine etiquette and respecting the dog's right to be treated with dignity.

• The first rule is the golden rule: If your child wouldn't like being screamed at, chased, poked, prodded, jumped on, or having his hair or ears pulled, he shouldn't do it to the dog. Keep an eye on things so you can step in when play gets rough or loud.

• Tell the child not to stare at the dog or bother him while he's eating or in his crate. In dog language, a stare is a challenge. If your dog has any aggressive tendencies, staring or the invasion of his territory could bring on a bite.

• Always supervise your child and dog. Dogs are not babysitters. No matter how trustworthy they seem, they should never be left alone with a baby or toddler.

• Include your children in the dog's care. A young child can fill up the water dish or food bowl, while an older one can be involved in the dog's grooming or training. Owning a dog without understanding any of the responsibilities required isn't much of a commitment.

If you've got a sled dog or draft breed, don't fight his instinct; instead, harness it and make it work for you. Let your dog pull you on skates or skis, or train him to pull a sled or dog-size cart. He'll get a workout, he won't be in trouble for pulling, and you'll have a new way to haul things.

☎ WHEN TO CALL THE VET

This type of behavior usually doesn't require any veterinary attention.

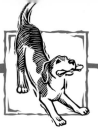

Where to Learn More

There are lots of knowledgeable sources for just about everything you want to know about dogs, from purebred registries and national, regional, and local breed clubs to training clubs, humane societies, and even World Wide Web sites.

Whatever your needs or interests, it's likely you'll find a dog group for you. The following list, while not complete, will help you find what you're looking for, whether it's a Golden Retriever breed club or a veterinary chiropractor.

ALTERNATIVE VETERINARY MEDICINE

American Holistic Veterinary Medical Association
2214 Old Emmorton Road
Bel Air, MD 21015
(410) 569-0795
Web site: http://www.altvetmed.com

American Veterinary Chiropractic Association
623 Main Street
Hillsdale, IL 61257
(309) 658-2920
E-mail: AmVetChiro@aol.com

International Veterinary Acupuncture Society
PO Box 2074
Nedorlund, CO 80466
(303) 258-3767

National Center for Homeopathy
801 North Fairfax Street, Suite 306
Alexandria, VA 22314
(703) 548-7790
Web site: http://homeopathic.org

 ## ANIMAL PROTECTION

American Humane Association
63 Inverness Drive East
Englewood, CO 80112-5117
(303) 792-9900

The Humane Animal Rescue Team
PO Box 920
Fillmore, CA 93016
(805) 524-4542

Humane Society of the United States
2100 L Street NW
Washington, DC 20037
(202) 452-1100
Web site: http://www.hsus.org

 BEHAVIOR AND TRAINING

American College of Veterinary Behaviorists
College of Veterinary Medicine
University of Georgia
Athens, Georgia 30602
(706) 542-8343

American Veterinary Society of Animal Behavior
Animal Behavior Consultations
4820 Rainbow Boulevard
Westwood, KS 66205
(913) 362-2512

The National Association of Dog Obedience Instructors (NADOI)
Attn: Corresponding Secretary
729 Grapevine Highway, Suite 369
Hurst, TX 76054

 PET LOSS SUPPORT HOTLINE

CALIFORNIA

University of California-Davis
School of Veterinary Medicine
Davis, CA 95616
(916) 752-4200
(916) 752-3602 to order free brochures
☺ Hours: 6:30 p.m. to 9:30 p.m. Pacific time, Monday through Friday.

Where to Learn More

COLORADO

Colorado State University Veterinary Teaching Hospital
"Changes" Support for People and Pets Program
300 W. Drake Road
Fort Collins, CO 80523
(970) 491-1242
⊙ Hours: 9:00 a.m. to 5:00 p.m., Mountain time, Tuesday, Thursday,
and Friday; 9:00 a.m. to 12:00 p.m., Mountain time, Wednesday.

FLORIDA

University of Florida
College of Veterinary Medicine
Box 100124
Gainesville, FL 32610
(904) 392-4700; then dial 1 and 4080
⊙ Hours: 7 p.m. to 9 p.m., Eastern time, Monday through Friday.

ILLINOIS

Chicago Veterinary Medical Association
Riser Animal Hospital
5335 West Touhy
Skokie, IL 60077
(630) 603-3994
⊙ Hours: 7 p.m. to 9 p.m., Central time, Monday through Friday.

MASSACHUSETTS

Tufts University
School of Veterinary Medicine
200 Westboro Road
North Grafton, MA 01536
(508) 839-7966
⊙ Hours: 6 p.m. to 9 p.m., Eastern time, Monday through Friday.

Michigan State University
College of Veterinary Medicine
A135 East Fee Hall
East Lansing, MI 48824
(517) 432-2696
☉ Hours: 6:30 p.m. to 9:30 p.m. Eastern time, Tuesday through
  Thursday.

 PUREBRED REGISTRIES/BREED CLUBS

American Kennel Club
51 Madison Avenue
New York, NY 10010
(212) 696-8200

States Kennel Club
PO Box 389
Hattiesburg, MS 39403-0389
(601) 583-8345

United Kennel Club
100 East Kilgore Road
Kalamazoo, MI 49002
(616) 343-9020

 TATTOO, TAG, AND MICROCHIP
REGISTRIES

AKC Companion Animal Recovery
5580 Centerview Drive, Suite 250
Raleigh, NC 27606-3394
(800) 252-7894
E-mail: found@akc.org

Identipet
74 Hoyt Street
Darien, Connecticut 06820
(800) 243-9147

InfoPET
415 West Travelers Trail
Burnsville, MN 55337
(800) INFOPET

National Dog Registry (NDR)
PO Box 116
Woodstock, NY 12498
(800) NDR-DOGS

Schering-Plough Animal Health
Attn: HomeAgain
Schering-Plough Liberty Hall
1095 Morris Avenue
Union, NJ 07083-1982
(800) 521-5767

 WORLD WIDE WEB SITES

Acme Pet
http://www.acmepet.com
Dog guide provides links to sites on activities, breeds, articles, health, humor, publications, and more.

The American Kennel Club
http://www.akc.org
Information on breeds, events, registration statistics, and choosing a breed. Provides links to breed club and breed rescue sites.

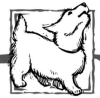

INDEX

Index